Low FODMAP Diet for Beginners

A Comprehensive Guide to Supporting Digestive Health with Easy and Tasty Recipes

Sophia Harper

Disclaimer

The information provided in this book is for educational and informational purposes only and is not intended as a substitute for professional medical advice, diagnosis, or treatment. Always consult your physician, registered dietitian, or other qualified healthcare provider before making significant changes to your diet or lifestyle, especially if you have a medical condition, are pregnant, or are taking medications.

While every effort has been made to ensure the accuracy of the information presented, the author and publisher make no representations or warranties of any kind regarding the completeness, accuracy, or applicability of the content. Any reliance you place on the information provided in this book is strictly at your own risk.

The author and publisher disclaim any liability for any direct, indirect, or consequential loss or damage arising from the use of the material contained in this book.

Dedication

To all those seeking better health and a vibrant life, this book is for you. May it inspire positive changes, bring comfort, and help you on your journey toward wellness.

Table of Contents

Introduction

If you've picked up this book, chances are you're searching for relief from digestive discomfort or looking for answers to unexplained symptoms like bloating, cramping, or irregular bowel movements. First, let me say—you're not alone. Digestive issues can be frustrating, confusing, and sometimes overwhelming. But here's the good news: with the right tools and understanding, you can take control of your health and start feeling better. That's exactly what this book is here to help you do.

The low FODMAP diet is a scientifically proven approach that has helped countless individuals manage conditions like irritable bowel syndrome (IBS) and other gut-related disorders. It's designed to reduce symptoms by identifying and limiting certain types of carbohydrates that can be hard for some people to digest. But don't worry—you won't have to say goodbye to delicious, satisfying meals. With a little guidance and preparation, you'll find this journey not only manageable but also rewarding.

This book is your step-by-step guide to understanding and implementing the low FODMAP diet. Whether you're just starting out or looking for practical advice to make the process easier, you'll find everything you need right here.

Why This Book Matters

For those living with IBS or other digestive challenges, everyday life can feel unpredictable. Social gatherings, workdays, and even meals at home can become stressful when you're unsure what will trigger discomfort. This book was created with you in mind—to provide clear, actionable solutions that will help you take back control.

Instead of wading through endless information online or feeling lost in complicated medical jargon, you'll find this book is written in plain, relatable language. It's designed to simplify the process, so you can focus on what really matters: your health and well-being.

What You'll Gain

By the time you finish this book, you'll have:

- A clear understanding of what FODMAPs are and how they affect your digestive system.

- A step-by-step plan to implement the low FODMAP diet, including guidance on the elimination, reintroduction, and personalization phases.

- Tools for meal planning, grocery shopping, and dining out with confidence.

- A collection of easy, delicious recipes that are gut-friendly and perfect for everyday life.

- Solutions for common challenges, so you can stay motivated and on track.

Most importantly, you'll gain the knowledge and confidence to make choices that support your health. You don't have to live in discomfort or feel like your gut is in charge—this book is here to help you regain control and live a life free from digestive distress.

A Supportive Journey Ahead

As you move through the chapters, think of this book as your companion. It's here to guide you, support you, and cheer you on every step of the way. Remember, small steps lead to big changes. You've already taken the first one by opening this book—let's take the next ones together.

Chapter 1

Understanding the Low FODMAP Diet

If you've ever experienced uncomfortable bloating, gas, or digestive distress after a meal, you're not alone. For many people, the culprit lies in a group of carbohydrates known as FODMAPs. Understanding these compounds and how they interact with your digestive system is the first step to finding relief and reclaiming control of your gut health.

What Are FODMAPs?

FODMAPs is an acronym that stands for **Fermentable Oligosaccharides, Disaccharides, Monosaccharides, and Polyols**—a mouthful, we know! But what does that mean in everyday terms? These are types of short-chain carbohydrates and sugar alcohols found in a variety of foods. For some people, these compounds are poorly absorbed in the small intestine, leading to fermentation by gut bacteria and the production of gas.

Here's a breakdown of the FODMAP categories:

- **Oligosaccharides**: Found in foods like wheat, onions, and garlic.

- **Disaccharides**: Lactose is the main disaccharide, found in milk and dairy products.

- **Monosaccharides**: Fructose is the key player here, found in high concentrations in fruits like apples, pears, and honey.

- **Polyols**: Sugar alcohols like sorbitol and mannitol, found in stone fruits, artificial sweeteners, and some vegetables.

High-FODMAP Foods and Their Effects

Here are some examples of high-FODMAP foods that may trigger symptoms in sensitive individuals:

- **Fruits**: Apples, watermelon, and cherries.

- **Vegetables**: Cauliflower, Brussels sprouts, and asparagus.

- **Dairy**: Milk, soft cheeses, and yogurt.

- **Legumes**: Lentils, chickpeas, and black beans.

- **Sweeteners**: Sorbitol and xylitol (often found in sugar-free gum and candy).

For individuals with conditions like IBS, consuming these foods can lead to symptoms such as bloating, gas, diarrhea, or constipation. This happens because the unabsorbed FODMAPs draw water into the gut and are fermented by bacteria, producing gas that causes discomfort.

The Role of FODMAPs in Digestive Health

In a healthy digestive system, FODMAPs may pass through without issue. However, for those with a sensitive gut, these compounds can become problematic. The symptoms they trigger can disrupt daily life, making it difficult to enjoy meals or socialize without worry.

Who Can Benefit from the Low FODMAP Diet?

The low FODMAP diet is particularly effective for managing **irritable bowel syndrome (IBS)**. It can also be helpful for other conditions, such as:

- **Inflammatory Bowel Disease (IBD)**: While not a cure, it may reduce symptoms during flare-ups.

- **Functional Gastrointestinal Disorders**: These include conditions where the structure of the digestive system appears normal but symptoms persist.

- **Small Intestinal Bacterial Overgrowth (SIBO)**: Some evidence suggests it may alleviate symptoms by reducing fermentable substrates for bacteria.

The Science Behind the Diet

The low FODMAP diet was developed by researchers at Monash University in Australia and is supported by a growing body of evidence. Studies have consistently shown its effectiveness in reducing symptoms of IBS, with some reporting improvement in up to 75% of individuals who follow the diet.

The diet works in three stages:

1. **Elimination**: Temporarily removing high-FODMAP foods to identify triggers.

2. **Reintroduction**: Gradually testing individual FODMAPs to determine personal tolerance levels.

3. **Personalization**: Creating a sustainable diet tailored to your unique needs and preferences.

The low FODMAP diet isn't about deprivation—it's about understanding your body and making choices that support your health. By identifying and managing your triggers, you can reduce uncomfortable symptoms and enjoy food with confidence again.

Chapter 2

Getting Started with the Low FODMAP Diet

Embarking on a new dietary journey can feel a bit overwhelming, but the good news is that you're not alone. With the right tools, mindset, and support, you can successfully navigate the low FODMAP diet and discover the foods that work best for your body. This chapter is your step-by-step guide to getting started, building confidence, and staying motivated along the way.

The Three Phases of the Low FODMAP Diet

The low FODMAP diet is designed as a three-phase process that helps you identify your personal triggers and build a sustainable way of eating. Let's break it down:

1. Elimination Phase

This is the starting point of your journey. In this phase, you'll temporarily remove all high-FODMAP foods from your diet. The goal is to give your digestive system a break and observe whether your symptoms improve.

- **Duration**: Typically lasts 4-6 weeks.
- **Key Tips**:
    o Focus on the many delicious low-FODMAP foods available.
    o Keep a food and symptom journal to track your progress.
    o Plan meals and snacks in advance to avoid feeling stuck.

2. Reintroduction Phase

Once your symptoms have stabilized, it's time to reintroduce high-FODMAP foods one at a time. This phase helps you determine which specific FODMAPs you tolerate well and which ones cause symptoms.

- **How It Works**:
    o Test one food at a time over several days.
    o Start with a small portion and gradually increase it.
    o Take notes on how your body reacts.
- **Key Tips**:
    o Be patient—this phase can take a few months.
    o Celebrate small victories as you identify safe foods.

3. Personalization Phase

This is the final phase, where you create a long-term diet tailored to your unique needs. You'll combine the foods you tolerate well with occasional indulgences in foods that may be less gut-friendly but are worth it for special occasions.

- **Goal**: Strike a balance between managing symptoms and enjoying a variety of foods.

- **Key Tips**:
    - Listen to your body and adjust as needed.
    - Experiment with recipes to keep meals exciting.
    - Remember, the diet is flexible and meant to adapt to your life.

Preparing for Success

Getting started with the low FODMAP diet isn't just about the foods you eat—it's also about your mindset and preparation. Here's how to set yourself up for success:

1. Shift Your Mindset

Think of this diet as an experiment, not a life sentence. It's an opportunity to learn about your body and take charge of your health.

2. Set Realistic Goals

- **Short-Term Goals**: Focus on completing each phase step by step.
- **Long-Term Goals**: Aim for better symptom management and improved quality of life.

3. Stock Your Kitchen

- Remove high-FODMAP foods that might tempt you during the elimination phase.
- Stock up on low-FODMAP staples like rice, potatoes, chicken, eggs, and lactose-free dairy.

4. Plan Ahead

- Create a list of go-to meals and snacks that are easy to prepare.
- Use meal planning to save time and reduce stress.

When to Consult a Professional

While the low FODMAP diet can be incredibly effective, it's always a good idea to seek guidance from a healthcare provider or dietitian, especially if:

- You're unsure where to start or feel overwhelmed.
- You have additional dietary restrictions or medical conditions.
- You want personalized advice tailored to your lifestyle.

Working with a professional can help you avoid common pitfalls, stay on track, and ensure you're meeting your nutritional needs.

Building Confidence and Overcoming Challenges

Starting any new diet can come with its challenges, but you've got this! Here are a few tips to keep you motivated:

- **Focus on Progress, Not Perfection**: If you accidentally eat a high-FODMAP food, don't panic. It's all part of the learning process.

- **Lean on Support**: Connect with others who are on the same journey. Online forums, social media groups, and friends can encourage.

- **Celebrate Small Wins**: Every time you try a new recipe, discover a safe food, or notice an improvement in your symptoms, take a moment to celebrate.

The low FODMAP diet is a journey toward better health and understanding your body. By approaching it step by step, preparing thoughtfully, and seeking support when needed, you'll build the confidence and skills to manage your symptoms and embrace a diet that works for you.

Chapter 3

Essential Ingredients for a Low FODMAP Pantry

Starting the low FODMAP diet can feel like a big change, but with the right ingredients in your kitchen, you'll be ready to tackle it with confidence. This chapter will help you stock a pantry full of essentials, find suitable substitutions for high-FODMAP foods, and choose products that fit seamlessly into your diet. With these tips, you'll be prepared to whip up delicious, gut-friendly meals without the stress.

Stocking Your Kitchen: Must-Have Low-FODMAP Staples

Building a low-FODMAP pantry begins with choosing the right basics. Here's a list of essentials that will serve as the foundation of your meals:

Grains and Starches

- **Rice**: White, brown, basmati, or jasmine.

- **Gluten-Free Bread**: Check labels to ensure no high-FODMAP ingredients like inulin or high-fructose corn syrup.

- **Gluten-Free Pasta**: Made from rice, corn, or quinoa.

- **Potatoes**: All types are low-FODMAP when prepared without high-FODMAP toppings.

- **Oats**: Ensure they are certified gluten-free.

Proteins

- **Chicken, Turkey, and Fish**: Fresh, unprocessed options are naturally low-FODMAP.

- **Eggs**: A versatile and easy-to-digest protein source.

- **Firm Tofu**: Look for plain tofu without added seasonings.

- **Lactose-Free Dairy**: Milk, yogurt, and cheese options specifically labeled as lactose-free.

Fruits and Vegetables

- **Low-FODMAP Vegetables**: Zucchini, spinach, carrots, cucumbers, and bell peppers.

- **Low-FODMAP Fruits**: Oranges, strawberries, blueberries, bananas (firm), and kiwi.

- **Canned Tomatoes**: Look for plain, no-onion or garlic-added versions.

Pantry Basics

- **Oils and Vinegars**: Olive oil, canola oil, and balsamic vinegar (in small amounts).

- **Spices and Herbs**: Basil, oregano, thyme, and paprika (avoid garlic and onion powders).

- **Stocks and Broths**: Choose low-FODMAP options or make your own.

Low-FODMAP Food Substitutes

When transitioning to a low FODMAP diet, finding replacements for high-FODMAP foods is key. Here are some swaps to make your favorite meals work for your new diet:

16

Dairy Alternatives

- **Replace Milk** with lactose-free milk, almond milk (unsweetened), or coconut milk (from a carton).

- **Replace Cream** with lactose-free cream or canned coconut cream in small amounts.

- **Replace Yogurt** with lactose-free yogurt or plain coconut yogurt.

Sweeteners

- **Avoid** high-FODMAP sweeteners like honey, high-fructose corn syrup, and agave.

- **Use** maple syrup, table sugar, or stevia instead.

Garlic and Onion

- **Replace Garlic** with garlic-infused oil (made by steeping garlic in oil and then discarding it).

- **Replace Onion** with the green tops of scallions or leeks, which are low-FODMAP.

Grains and Baked Goods

- **Replace Wheat Flour** with gluten-free flour blends or rice flour.

- **Replace Regular Bread** with certified gluten-free bread.

Recommended Low-FODMAP-Friendly Brands

Finding the right products can simplify your journey. Here are some trusted brands that cater to low-FODMAP eaters:

- **Fody Foods**: Offers low-FODMAP sauces, dressings, and snacks.

- **Casa de Santé**: Known for its seasonings and meal kits.

- **Lactaid**: Provides a range of lactose-free dairy products.

- **Barilla**: Gluten-free pasta options that are low-FODMAP.

- **Enjoy Life**: Certified gluten-free and allergen-friendly snacks.

Label Reading Tips

Understanding food labels is crucial for avoiding hidden FODMAPs. Here's how to shop smarter:

1. **Look for Hidden Ingredients**

   o Watch out for high-FODMAP additives like inulin, high-fructose corn syrup, and polyols (e.g., sorbitol, mannitol).

2. **Choose Simple Ingredients**

   o Opt for products with short ingredient lists and minimal processing.

3. **Check for Certifications**

   o Look for gluten-free and lactose-free labels, but always verify other ingredients.

4. **Beware of Natural Flavors**

o   These can sometimes include onion or garlic. Double-check with the manufacturer if you're unsure.

Stocking a low-FODMAP pantry is all about preparation and smart choices. With the right staples, substitutions, and brands, you'll have everything you need to cook confidently and enjoy meals that support your digestive health. Taking the time to read labels and explore new ingredients will make your journey not only manageable but also rewarding.

Chapter 4

Meal Planning and Preparation

Adopting a low FODMAP diet doesn't mean sacrificing convenience or variety in your meals. With a little planning and preparation, you can enjoy delicious, gut-friendly meals that fit your lifestyle, whether you're at home, at work, or on the go. This chapter is packed with practical tips to make your low FODMAP journey smooth and stress-free.

Creating Weekly Meal Plans

Meal planning is a powerful tool to save time, reduce stress, and ensure you stick to your low FODMAP diet. Here's how to get started:

Step 1: Assess Your Week

Take a few minutes to review your schedule. Identify busy days when you might need quick meals or snacks and plan accordingly.

Step 2: Build Your Menu

- **Breakfasts**: Choose simple, repeatable options like overnight oats made with lactose-free milk or scrambled eggs with spinach.

- **Lunches**: Plan balanced meals with protein, low-FODMAP veggies, and a small serving of low-FODMAP grains.

- **Dinners**: Incorporate variety by rotating recipes like grilled chicken with roasted zucchini or baked salmon with mashed potatoes.

- **Snacks**: Include easy options such as low-FODMAP fruits, lactose-free yogurt, or rice cakes with peanut butter.

Step 3: Write Your Shopping List

Based on your menu, create a detailed shopping list. Stick to low-FODMAP staples and double-check labels for hidden high-FODMAP ingredients.

Step 4: Prep Ahead

Set aside time each week to wash, chop, and portion ingredients. Having everything ready to go makes cooking much quicker.

Batch Cooking Tips

Batch cooking is a lifesaver for busy weeks. It allows you to prepare multiple meals in advance, so you always have something low FODMAP-friendly on hand.

Strategy 1: Cook in Bulk

- Prepare large portions of soups, stews, or casseroles that can be divided into individual servings and frozen for later.

- Roast a big batch of vegetables and store them in airtight containers for easy side dishes throughout the week.

Strategy 2: Mix and Match

- Cook versatile staples like grilled chicken, quinoa, or roasted sweet potatoes. Use them as building blocks for different meals, such as salads, wraps, or stir-fries.

Strategy 3: Freeze Smart

- Store meals in labeled, portion-sized containers. This makes it easy to grab and reheat a meal without guessing what's inside.

- Use freezer-safe bags to save space and keep ingredients fresh.

Strategy 4: Use Your Slow Cooker or Instant Pot

- These appliances are perfect for hands-off cooking. Make dishes like pulled pork or vegetable soup that can cook while you focus on other tasks.

On-the-Go Meal Ideas

Sticking to a low FODMAP diet while at work, school, or traveling can feel challenging, but with a little preparation, it's entirely doable.

Work or School

- **Salads in a Jar**: Layer low-FODMAP ingredients like spinach, grilled chicken, and quinoa. Keep the dressing in a separate container to avoid sogginess.

- **Wraps and Sandwiches**: Use gluten-free wraps or bread with fillings like turkey, lettuce, and lactose-free cheese.

- **Snack Packs**: Assemble a mix of almonds, low-FODMAP fruits, and rice crackers for quick energy.

Travel

- **Pack Ahead**: Prepare meals like grilled chicken with roasted veggies in portable containers.

- **Low-FODMAP Snacks**: Carry shelf-stable options like rice cakes, lactose-free cheese sticks, or bananas.

- **Research Restaurants**: If dining out, check menus online and call ahead to ask about low FODMAP options.

Emergency Options

Always keep a stash of low-FODMAP snacks in your bag, car, or desk drawer. This ensures you'll have something to eat even in unexpected situations.

Planning and preparation are essential tools for succeeding on a low FODMAP diet. By creating weekly meal plans, embracing batch cooking, and packing smart on-the-go meals, you'll not only save time and reduce stress but also ensure you have access to satisfying and gut-friendly food no matter where life takes you.

Chapter 5

Breakfast Recipes

Start your day right with these delicious and easy-to-make low FODMAP breakfast recipes. Each one is designed to support your digestive health while giving you the energy you need to kickstart your morning. These recipes are not only gentle on your gut but also packed with flavor and nutrients to fuel your day.

Scrambled Eggs with Spinach and Feta

A protein-packed, savory breakfast that's quick to make and satisfying.

Estimated Meal Time: 10 minutes

Ingredients:

- 2 large eggs
- 1 cup fresh spinach, chopped
- 2 tbsp crumbled feta cheese (lactose-free)
- Salt and pepper to taste
- 1 tsp olive oil or butter

Cooking Method:

1. Heat olive oil or butter in a pan over medium heat.
2. Add spinach and sauté for 1-2 minutes until wilted.
3. In a bowl, whisk eggs, salt, and pepper. Pour into the pan with spinach.
4. Cook for 2-3 minutes, stirring occasionally, until eggs are scrambled and cooked through.
5. Top with crumbled feta cheese and serve immediately.

Nutritional Facts (per serving):

- Calories: 290 | Protein: 18g | Carbs: 3g | Fat: 22g | Fiber: 2g

Substitution Variations:

- Use goat cheese instead of feta for a different flavor.
- Add fresh herbs like parsley or chives for extra freshness.

Portion Control:

- One serving equals the entire recipe, providing a balanced meal with protein and healthy fats.

Pro Tips:

- For a creamier texture, add a tablespoon of lactose-free milk when whisking the eggs.
- Serve with gluten-free toast for a more filling meal.

Quinoa Porridge with Strawberries

A warm, comforting breakfast that's packed with protein and fiber to keep you full.

Estimated Meal Time: 20 minutes

Ingredients:

- 1/2 cup quinoa
- 1 cup water or unsweetened almond milk
- 1/4 cup strawberries, sliced
- 1 tbsp chia seeds
- 1 tsp maple syrup (optional)
- 1/2 tsp vanilla extract

Cooking Method:

1. Rinse quinoa under cold water.
2. In a pot, bring water or almond milk to a boil. Add quinoa and reduce to a simmer. Cover and cook for 15-18 minutes until quinoa is soft and the liquid is absorbed.

3. Stir in chia seeds, vanilla extract, and maple syrup.

4. Top with sliced strawberries and serve.

Nutritional Facts (per serving):

- Calories: 220 | Protein: 6g | Carbs: 38g | Fat: 6g | Fiber: 6g

Substitution Variations:

- Use coconut milk for a richer, creamier texture.

- Add other low FODMAP fruits like blueberries or kiwi for variety.

Portion Control:

- One serving equals about 1 cup of quinoa porridge, providing a satisfying breakfast that's high in fiber.

Pro Tips:

- Make a big batch of quinoa in advance and store in the fridge for up to 3 days.

- Add a sprinkle of cinnamon for extra flavor.

Oatmeal with Blueberries and Almond Butter

A hearty oatmeal that's easy to prepare and great for gut health.

Estimated Meal Time: 15 minutes

Ingredients:

- 1 cup rolled oats
- 2 cups unsweetened almond milk
- 1/4 cup blueberries
- 1 tbsp almond butter
- 1 tsp honey (optional)

Cooking Method:

1. In a saucepan, combine oats and almond milk. Cook over medium heat, stirring occasionally, for 5–7 minutes until oats are tender.
2. Stir in almond butter and mix until well combined.
3. Top with blueberries and a drizzle of honey if desired.

Nutritional Facts (per serving):

- Calories: 280 | Protein: 8g | Carbs: 36g | Fat: 14g | Fiber: 6g

Substitution Variations:

- Swap almond butter for peanut butter or sunflower seed butter.
- Use strawberries or raspberries instead of blueberries for a different flavor.

Portion Control:

- One serving equals about 1½ cups of oatmeal, which is a hearty breakfast providing balanced nutrition.

Pro Tips:

- Prepare the oats the night before for a quicker breakfast in the morning.
- Sprinkle with chia seeds or flaxseeds for added fiber.

Chia Seed Pudding with Coconut Milk

A simple, make-ahead breakfast that's great for busy mornings.

Estimated Meal Time: 5 minutes (plus overnight chilling)

Ingredients:

- 1/4 cup chia seeds
- 1 cup unsweetened coconut milk
- 1 tsp vanilla extract
- 1 tbsp maple syrup (optional)

Cooking Method:

1. In a bowl, combine chia seeds, coconut milk, vanilla extract, and maple syrup.
2. Stir well to combine and ensure the chia seeds are fully submerged.
3. Cover and refrigerate for at least 4 hours or overnight.
4. Top with your favorite low-FODMAP fruit before serving.

Nutritional Facts (per serving):

- Calories: 180 | Protein: 6g | Carbs: 12g | Fat: 14g | Fiber: 10g

Substitution Variations:

- Use almond milk or oat milk if you prefer a different base.
- Add toppings like sliced strawberries, kiwi, or a sprinkle of shredded coconut.

Portion Control:

- One serving equals about 1/2 cup of chia pudding, providing a filling breakfast rich in fiber and healthy fats.

Pro Tips:

- Make the pudding the night before for a hassle-free breakfast.
- If you prefer a sweeter flavor, add more maple syrup or a dash of cinnamon.

Low FODMAP Banana Pancakes

Fluffy and light pancakes made with ripe bananas and gluten-free flour, perfect for a relaxing morning.

Estimated Meal Time: 20 minutes

Ingredients:

- 1 ripe banana, mashed
- 2 eggs
- 1/2 cup gluten-free flour
- 1 tsp baking powder
- 1/4 tsp cinnamon
- 1/4 tsp vanilla extract
- 1 tbsp lactose-free milk

Cooking Method:

1. In a bowl, whisk together the mashed banana, eggs, gluten-free flour, baking powder, cinnamon, vanilla extract, and lactose-free milk.
2. Heat a non-stick pan over medium heat and lightly grease it with oil or butter.
3. Pour the pancake batter into the pan, forming small circles. Cook for 2-3 minutes on each side until golden brown.
4. Serve with your favorite low-FODMAP syrup or fresh fruit.

Nutritional Facts (per serving):

- Calories: 180 | Protein: 6g | Carbs: 24g | Fat: 8g | Fiber: 3g

Substitution Variations:

- Use coconut flour instead of gluten-free flour for a different texture.
- Add blueberries or strawberries to the batter for extra flavor.

Portion Control:

- One serving equals 2-3 pancakes, depending on size, providing a balanced breakfast with carbs and protein.

Pro Tips:

- For fluffier pancakes, let the batter rest for a few minutes before cooking.
- Freeze extra pancakes for a quick breakfast option later.

Greek Yogurt with Maple Syrup and Walnuts

A creamy, indulgent breakfast that's quick to prepare and full of healthy fats and protein.

Estimated Meal Time: 5 minutes

Ingredients:

- 1/2 cup plain Greek yogurt (lactose-free)
- 1 tbsp maple syrup
- 1 tbsp chopped walnuts
- A pinch of cinnamon (optional)

Cooking Method:

1. In a bowl, place the Greek yogurt and drizzle with maple syrup.
2. Top with chopped walnuts and a sprinkle of cinnamon if desired.
3. Serve immediately and enjoy.

Nutritional Facts (per serving):

- Calories: 250 | Protein: 12g | Carbs: 22g | Fat: 16g | Fiber: 2g

Substitution Variations:

- Use almonds or pecans instead of walnuts.
- Add fresh berries like blueberries or raspberries for extra antioxidants.

Portion Control:

- One serving equals 1/2 cup of Greek yogurt, providing a filling breakfast with protein and healthy fats.

Pro Tips:

- Use coconut yogurt if you prefer a dairy-free option.
- Add a drizzle of honey for extra sweetness.

Avocado Toast with Gluten-Free Bread

A classic breakfast option that's simple, satisfying, and packed with healthy fats.

Estimated Meal Time: 10 minutes

Ingredients:

- 1 slice gluten-free bread
- 1/2 ripe avocado
- Salt and pepper to taste
- Red pepper flakes or fresh herbs (optional)

Cooking Method:

1. Toast the slice of gluten-free bread to your preference.
2. Mash the avocado with a fork and spread it evenly on the toast.
3. Season with salt, pepper, and red pepper flakes or fresh herbs if desired.
4. Serve immediately for a quick, nutritious breakfast.

Nutritional Facts (per serving):

- Calories: 250 | Protein: 4g | Carbs: 20g | Fat: 20g | Fiber: 9g

Substitution Variations:

- Add a poached egg on top for extra protein.
- Sprinkle with sesame seeds or pumpkin seeds for added texture.

Portion Control:

- One serving equals 1 slice of avocado toast, making for a light yet fulfilling meal.

Pro Tips:

- Use gluten-free bread that's high in fiber for added benefits.
- For a more filling meal, serve with a side of fruit.

Rice Cakes with Peanut Butter and Banana

A quick and satisfying breakfast option that combines healthy fats, protein, and fiber.

Estimated Meal Time: 5 minutes

Ingredients:

- 2 rice cakes
- 2 tbsp peanut butter (check for no added sugar)
- 1 small banana, sliced

Cooking Method:

1. Spread peanut butter evenly on each rice cake.
2. Top with banana slices and enjoy immediately.

Nutritional Facts (per serving):

- Calories: 300 | Protein: 9g | Carbs: 36g | Fat: 16g | Fiber: 5g

Substitution Variations:

- Use almond butter instead of peanut butter.
- Swap the banana for strawberries or kiwi for a fresh twist.

Portion Control:

- One serving equals 2 rice cakes, providing a balanced and satisfying breakfast.

Pro Tips:

- Choose brown rice cakes for extra fiber.
- If you prefer a sweeter touch, drizzle with a bit of honey or maple syrup.

Smoothie with Spinach, Pineapple, and Lactose-Free Yogurt

A refreshing, nutrient-packed smoothie that's perfect for busy mornings.

Estimated Meal Time: 5 minutes

Ingredients:

- 1 cup fresh spinach
- 1/2 cup pineapple chunks (fresh or frozen)
- 1/2 cup lactose-free yogurt
- 1/2 cup water or unsweetened almond milk
- Ice cubes (optional)

Cooking Method:

1. Combine spinach, pineapple, yogurt, and almond milk in a blender.
2. Blend until smooth and creamy, adding ice cubes for a chilled texture if desired.
3. Pour into a glass and serve immediately.

Nutritional Facts (per serving):

- Calories: 180 | Protein: 6g | Carbs: 34g | Fat: 2g | Fiber: 4g

Substitution Variations:

- Use coconut yogurt for a dairy-free smoothie.

- Swap pineapple for mango or berries for different flavors.

Portion Control:

- One serving equals one smoothie, providing a light but nutrient-rich breakfast.

Pro Tips:

- Add a tablespoon of chia seeds or flaxseeds for extra fiber and omega-3s.

- For a more filling smoothie, add a scoop of protein powder.

Omelette with Bell Peppers and Zucchini

A veggie-filled omelette that's packed with flavor and protein to start your day off right.

Estimated Meal Time: 10 minutes

Ingredients:

- 2 eggs
- 1/4 cup bell peppers, diced
- 1/4 cup zucchini, diced
- 1 tbsp olive oil or butter
- Salt and pepper to taste

Cooking Method:

1. Heat olive oil or butter in a pan over medium heat.
2. Add diced bell peppers and zucchini, and sauté for 2-3 minutes until softened.
3. Whisk eggs with salt and pepper, then pour into the pan over the vegetables.
4. Cook for another 2-3 minutes until the eggs are set. Fold the omelette and serve.

Nutritional Facts (per serving):

- Calories: 220 | Protein: 14g | Carbs: 6g | Fat: 16g | Fiber: 2g

Substitution Variations:

- Use spinach or mushrooms instead of zucchini for a different veggie mix.

- Add a sprinkle of lactose-free cheese for extra flavor.

Portion Control:

- One serving equals one omelette, providing a satisfying and balanced meal.

Pro Tips:

- Add fresh herbs like chives or parsley to enhance the flavor.

- Serve with a side of gluten-free toast for a fuller meal.

Low FODMAP Overnight Oats with Almond Milk

A make-ahead breakfast that's ready when you are, packed with fiber and easy to digest.

Estimated Meal Time: 5 minutes (overnight preparation)

Ingredients:

- 1/2 cup rolled oats
- 1/2 cup unsweetened almond milk
- 1 tbsp chia seeds
- 1/2 tsp vanilla extract
- 1/4 tsp cinnamon
- 1/4 cup blueberries (fresh or frozen)

Cooking Method:

1. In a mason jar or airtight container, combine oats, almond milk, chia seeds, vanilla extract, and cinnamon.
2. Stir well, cover, and refrigerate overnight.
3. In the morning, top with fresh or frozen blueberries and enjoy!

Nutritional Facts (per serving):

- Calories: 220 | Protein: 6g | Carbs: 34g | Fat: 8g | Fiber: 9g

Substitution Variations:

- Swap blueberries for strawberries, raspberries, or kiwi.
- Add a handful of nuts or seeds for extra crunch.

Portion Control:

- One serving equals about 1½ cups of overnight oats, providing a balanced mix of fiber and healthy fats.

Pro Tips:

- Make several jars at once for a quick breakfast throughout the week.
- If you prefer a creamier texture, add more almond milk in the morning.

Scrambled Eggs with Fresh Herbs and Tomatoes

A simple, nutrient-packed breakfast that's full of flavor and easy to prepare.

Estimated Meal Time: 10 minutes

Ingredients:

- 2 eggs
- 1/4 cup cherry tomatoes, halved
- 1 tbsp fresh herbs (parsley, chives, or basil)
- 1 tbsp olive oil or butter
- Salt and pepper to taste

Cooking Method:

1. Heat olive oil or butter in a non-stick pan over medium heat.
2. Add the halved tomatoes and sauté for 2-3 minutes until softened.
3. Whisk the eggs with salt and pepper, then pour into the pan with tomatoes.
4. Stir gently until the eggs are fully cooked, then sprinkle with fresh herbs.
5. Serve immediately.

Nutritional Facts (per serving):

- Calories: 250 | Protein: 14g | Carbs: 6g | Fat: 18g | Fiber: 2g

Substitution Variations:

- Add spinach or bell peppers for extra veggies.
- Use lactose-free cheese for added richness.

Portion Control:

- One serving equals the scrambled eggs with a side of tomatoes, offering a filling, protein-rich breakfast.

Pro Tips:

- For fluffier scrambled eggs, add a splash of water or lactose-free milk while whisking.

- Pair with a side of gluten-free toast or rice cakes for a more substantial meal.

Buckwheat Pancakes with Strawberries

Delicious, nutty pancakes made from gluten-free buckwheat flour, perfect for a hearty breakfast.

Estimated Meal Time: 20 minutes

Ingredients:

- 1/2 cup buckwheat flour
- 1/4 tsp baking powder
- 1/4 tsp cinnamon
- 1 egg
- 1/2 cup unsweetened almond milk
- 1 tsp vanilla extract
- 1/4 cup strawberries, sliced
- 1 tbsp maple syrup (optional)

Cooking Method:

1. In a bowl, combine buckwheat flour, baking powder, and cinnamon.
2. In a separate bowl, whisk the egg, almond milk, and vanilla extract.
3. Combine the wet and dry ingredients to form a batter.
4. Heat a non-stick pan over medium heat and lightly grease it.
5. Pour the batter into the pan and cook each side for 2-3 minutes, or until golden brown.
6. Top with fresh strawberries and a drizzle of maple syrup if desired.

Nutritional Facts (per serving):

- Calories: 220 | Protein: 7g | Carbs: 30g | Fat: 8g | Fiber: 4g

Substitution Variations:

- Add blueberries or banana slices instead of strawberries.
- Use coconut milk for a richer flavor.

Portion Control:

- One serving equals 2-3 pancakes, providing a satisfying balance of carbs and protein.

Pro Tips:

- Make extra pancakes and freeze them for an easy breakfast option later in the week.
- Serve with a dollop of lactose-free yogurt for extra creaminess.

Baked Sweet Potato with Cinnamon and Walnuts

A warm, comforting breakfast that's rich in vitamins and fiber.

Estimated Meal Time: 40 minutes

Ingredients:

- 1 medium sweet potato
- 1 tbsp walnuts, chopped
- 1/2 tsp cinnamon
- 1 tsp maple syrup (optional)

Cooking Method:

1. Preheat the oven to 375°F (190°C).
2. Pierce the sweet potato with a fork and bake it for 30-40 minutes, or until soft.
3. Once baked, cut the sweet potato open and fluff with a fork.
4. Top with cinnamon, chopped walnuts, and a drizzle of maple syrup if desired.
5. Serve immediately.

Nutritional Facts (per serving):

- Calories: 250 | Protein: 4g | Carbs: 45g | Fat: 12g | Fiber: 7g

Substitution Variations:

- Use pecans or almonds instead of walnuts for variety.
- Add a dollop of lactose-free yogurt for extra creaminess.

Portion Control:

- One serving equals one medium baked sweet potato, offering a filling breakfast with complex carbs and healthy fats.

Pro Tips:

- Bake multiple sweet potatoes at once to have a quick, easy breakfast option ready for the next day.

- For a twist, sprinkle with nutmeg or ginger along with the cinnamon.

Low FODMAP Breakfast Burrito with Eggs and Spinach

A savory, protein-packed breakfast burrito that's perfect for an on-the-go meal.

Estimated Meal Time: 15 minutes

Ingredients:

- 1 gluten-free tortilla
- 2 eggs
- 1/4 cup spinach, chopped
- 1/4 cup lactose-free cheese (optional)
- 1 tbsp olive oil or butter
- Salt and pepper to taste

Cooking Method:

1. Heat olive oil or butter in a pan over medium heat.
2. Add spinach and sauté until wilted, about 1-2 minutes.
3. Whisk eggs with salt and pepper, then pour into the pan and scramble with the spinach.
4. Once the eggs are cooked, transfer them to the gluten-free tortilla.
5. Optionally, sprinkle with lactose-free cheese, then wrap up the tortilla and serve.

Nutritional Facts (per serving):

- Calories: 300 | Protein: 18g | Carbs: 18g | Fat: 18g | Fiber: 4g

Substitution Variations:

- Add bell peppers or zucchini for extra vegetables.
- Swap spinach for kale or arugula.

Portion Control:

- One serving equals one breakfast burrito, providing a satisfying combination of protein, carbs, and healthy fats.

Pro Tips:

- For an even quicker option, prepare the filling the night before and assemble the burrito in the morning.
- Serve with a side of fruit for extra nutrition.

Cottage Cheese with Blueberries and Chia Seeds

A light, protein-packed breakfast that's both refreshing and filling.

Estimated Meal Time: 5 minutes

Ingredients:

- 1/2 cup cottage cheese (lactose-free if needed)
- 1/4 cup fresh blueberries
- 1 tbsp chia seeds
- 1 tsp honey or maple syrup (optional)

Cooking Method:

1. In a bowl, combine the cottage cheese and chia seeds.
2. Top with fresh blueberries and drizzle with honey or maple syrup, if desired.
3. Serve immediately or refrigerate for later.

Nutritional Facts (per serving):

- Calories: 200 | Protein: 14g | Carbs: 15g | Fat: 12g | Fiber: 5g

Substitution Variations:

- Swap blueberries for raspberries or strawberries.
- Add a handful of nuts or seeds for extra crunch.

Portion Control:

- One serving equals about 1/2 cup cottage cheese, providing a healthy serving of protein and fiber.

Pro Tips:

- This is a great option for a quick breakfast or snack.

- Prepare the night before for an easy, grab-and-go breakfast.

Low FODMAP Muesli with Almond Milk

A hearty, no-cook breakfast that's perfect for busy mornings and packed with nutrients.

Estimated Meal Time: 5 minutes (overnight preparation)

Ingredients:

- 1/2 cup rolled oats
- 1/4 cup chopped nuts (almonds, walnuts, or pecans)
- 1/4 cup dried cranberries or raisins (low-FODMAP serving size)
- 1/2 cup unsweetened almond milk
- 1 tbsp chia seeds

Cooking Method:

1. In a jar or airtight container, combine oats, nuts, dried cranberries, chia seeds, and almond milk.
2. Stir well, cover, and refrigerate overnight.
3. In the morning, enjoy it cold, or heat it up if preferred.

Nutritional Facts (per serving):

- Calories: 300 | Protein: 8g | Carbs: 34g | Fat: 16g | Fiber: 9g

Substitution Variations:

- Use coconut milk or oat milk instead of almond milk.
- Replace cranberries with blueberries or strawberries for added freshness.

Portion Control:

- One serving equals about 1½ cups of muesli, offering a balanced combination of protein, fiber, and healthy fats.

Pro Tips:

- Make a batch for the week to save time in the morning.

- Add a dollop of lactose-free yogurt for extra creaminess and protein.

FODMAP-Friendly Breakfast Quesadilla with Turkey

A savory, protein-packed breakfast that's both filling and delicious, perfect for starting your day right.

Estimated Meal Time: 15 minutes

Ingredients:

- 1 gluten-free tortilla
- 2 oz turkey breast (deli-style, low-FODMAP)
- 1/4 cup lactose-free cheese, shredded
- 1 egg
- 1 tbsp olive oil or butter
- Salt and pepper to taste

Cooking Method:

1. Heat olive oil or butter in a pan over medium heat.
2. Crack the egg into the pan and scramble until fully cooked.
3. Lay the turkey breast on the gluten-free tortilla, then top with scrambled eggs and cheese.
4. Fold the tortilla and cook in the pan until golden and crispy on both sides.
5. Slice and serve immediately.

Nutritional Facts (per serving):

- Calories: 320 | Protein: 24g | Carbs: 18g | Fat: 20g | Fiber: 3g

Substitution Variations:

- Use chicken breast or ham instead of turkey.
- Add spinach or bell peppers for extra veggies.

Portion Control:

- One serving equals one quesadilla, providing a filling, protein-rich meal.

Pro Tips:

- Make it ahead and refrigerate for a quick breakfast option during the week.

- For extra flavor, add a dash of hot sauce or salsa on the side (ensure it's low-FODMAP).

Gluten-Free Banana Nut Muffins

A moist, sweet muffin that's perfect for breakfast or an on-the-go snack.

Estimated Meal Time: 30 minutes

Ingredients:

- 2 ripe bananas, mashed
- 1 ½ cups gluten-free flour blend
- 1 tsp baking soda
- 1/4 tsp cinnamon
- 1/4 tsp salt
- 2 eggs
- 1/4 cup maple syrup
- 1/4 cup walnut pieces (optional)
- 1/4 cup lactose-free yogurt

Cooking Method:

1. Preheat the oven to 350°F (175°C).
2. In a bowl, combine gluten-free flour, baking soda, cinnamon, and salt.
3. In a separate bowl, whisk the eggs, mashed bananas, maple syrup, and yogurt until smooth.
4. Fold in the dry ingredients until just combined.
5. Stir in walnut pieces if using.
6. Spoon the batter into a muffin tin lined with paper cups and bake for 18-20 minutes or until a toothpick comes out clean.
7. Let cool before serving.

Nutritional Facts (per muffin):

- Calories: 220 | Protein: 5g | Carbs: 30g | Fat: 10g | Fiber: 4g

Substitution Variations:

- Swap walnuts for pecans or almonds.

- Add chocolate chips for a sweet treat.

Portion Control:

- One serving equals one muffin, providing a balanced breakfast with healthy fats and natural sweetness.

Pro Tips:

- Make extra muffins and freeze them for a quick breakfast or snack.
- Enjoy with a hot cup of tea or coffee for the perfect morning pairing.

Poached Eggs on Rice Cakes with Spinach

A light, yet filling breakfast option that's easy to make and gluten-free.

Estimated Meal Time: 10 minutes

Ingredients:

- 2 eggs
- 2 rice cakes (plain or lightly salted)
- 1/4 cup spinach, sautéed
- Salt and pepper to taste

Cooking Method:

1. Poach the eggs to your desired level of doneness.
2. While the eggs cook, toast the rice cakes and sauté the spinach in a pan until wilted (about 2-3 minutes).
3. Top each rice cake with sautéed spinach, followed by a poached egg.
4. Sprinkle with salt and pepper, and serve immediately.

Nutritional Facts (per serving):

- Calories: 240 | Protein: 12g | Carbs: 22g | Fat: 14g | Fiber: 4g

Substitution Variations:

- Swap spinach for kale or arugula.

- Use avocado instead of rice cakes for a different texture.

Portion Control:

- One serving equals 2 poached eggs with rice cakes and spinach, providing a balanced mix of protein, fiber, and healthy fats.

Pro Tips:

- For extra protein, top with a sprinkle of lactose-free cheese or seeds.

- If you prefer a more filling breakfast, add a side of fruit or a small smoothie.

These breakfast recipes are designed to be easy, quick, and supportive of your journey on the low FODMAP diet. Enjoy every bite while knowing you're giving your body the nutrition it needs without triggering digestive issues.

Lunch Recipes

Enjoy a satisfying and nutritious lunch with these delicious low FODMAP recipes. Whether you're looking for a light salad, hearty bowl, or a flavorful wrap, each of these meals is designed to support your digestive health while keeping you energized and satisfied throughout the day. These recipes are easy to prepare and offer a variety of flavors, all while being gentle on your gut. Get ready to discover lunch ideas that are both healthy and full of taste!

Grilled Chicken Salad with Mixed Greens

A light yet filling salad with grilled chicken and fresh greens, perfect for a low FODMAP lunch.

Estimated Meal Time: 20 minutes

Ingredients:

- 1 boneless, skinless chicken breast
- 4 cups mixed greens (spinach, arugula, and lettuce)
- 1/4 cup sliced cucumber
- 1/4 cup cherry tomatoes, halved
- 1 tbsp olive oil
- 1 tbsp balsamic vinegar
- Salt and pepper to taste

Cooking Method:

1. Season the chicken breast with salt, pepper, and a drizzle of olive oil. Grill for 6-7 minutes on each side or until fully cooked.
2. While the chicken cooks, prepare the salad by combining the mixed greens, cucumber, and tomatoes in a bowl.
3. Slice the grilled chicken and add it to the salad.
4. Drizzle with balsamic vinegar and olive oil, then toss gently.
5. Serve immediately.

Nutritional Facts (per serving):

- Calories: 250 | Protein: 30g | Carbs: 8g | Fat: 14g | Fiber: 4g

Substitution Variations:

- Swap chicken for grilled turkey or tofu for a vegetarian option.
- Add a sprinkle of feta cheese or olives for extra flavor.

Portion Control:

- One serving includes one grilled chicken breast and a hearty portion of salad.

Pro Tips:

- Prep extra grilled chicken to use in salads or wraps throughout the week.
- Make a simple dressing with olive oil, lemon juice, and mustard for a low-FODMAP-friendly option.

Quinoa and Roasted Vegetable Bowl

A hearty, nutrient-dense bowl with quinoa and roasted veggies, perfect for a balanced lunch.

Estimated Meal Time: 30 minutes

Ingredients:

- 1 cup cooked quinoa
- 1 cup zucchini, diced
- 1 cup bell peppers, diced
- 1/2 cup carrots, sliced
- 1 tbsp olive oil
- 1 tsp dried oregano
- Salt and pepper to taste

Cooking Method:

1. Preheat your oven to 400°F (200°C).
2. Toss the zucchini, bell peppers, and carrots with olive oil, oregano, salt, and pepper. Spread them on a baking sheet.
3. Roast until vegetables are soft and gently browned, 20 to 25 minutes, turning halfway through.

4. Serve the roasted vegetables over a bed of cooked quinoa.

Nutritional Facts (per serving):

- Calories: 320 | Protein: 9g | Carbs: 45g | Fat: 12g | Fiber: 8g

Substitution Variations:

- Add roasted sweet potatoes or butternut squash for more flavor.

- Top with grilled chicken, tofu, or chickpeas for added protein.

Portion Control:

- One serving includes 1 cup of quinoa and roasted vegetables, offering a balanced meal.

Pro Tips:

- Make extra quinoa and roasted veggies for easy lunches during the week.

- Drizzle with a tahini dressing or low-FODMAP vinaigrette for extra flavor.

Turkey and Spinach Lettuce Wraps

A simple and fresh lunch idea, using lettuce as a low-FODMAP alternative to wraps.

Estimated Meal Time: 10 minutes

Ingredients:

- 4 large lettuce leaves (butter or Romaine lettuce)
- 4 oz sliced turkey breast (low-FODMAP)
- 1/2 cup spinach
- 1/4 cup shredded carrots
- 1 tbsp mustard or mayonnaise (low-FODMAP)

Cooking Method:

1. Lay the lettuce leaves flat on a plate.
2. Layer with sliced turkey, spinach, and shredded carrots.
3. Drizzle with mustard or mayonnaise, then fold the lettuce leaves around the fillings to create wraps.
4. Serve immediately.

Nutritional Facts (per serving):

- Calories: 200 | Protein: 24g | Carbs: 10g | Fat: 8g | Fiber: 3g

Substitution Variations:

- Swap turkey for chicken or ham.
- Add cucumber or avocado for extra crunch and creaminess.

Portion Control:

- One serving equals 4 wraps, providing a balanced protein and vegetable intake.

Pro Tips:

- These wraps are perfect for meal prep; simply pack the ingredients separately and assemble when ready to eat.
- Add a side of fruit or a handful of nuts for extra nutrients.

Low FODMAP Tuna Salad with Cucumber

A fresh and light tuna salad, made with cucumber and a simple dressing for a refreshing lunch.

Estimated Meal Time: 10 minutes

Ingredients:

- 1 can tuna in water, drained
- 1/2 cucumber, diced
- 1 tbsp olive oil
- 1 tbsp lemon juice
- Salt and pepper to taste

Cooking Method:

1. In a bowl, combine the tuna, diced cucumber, olive oil, and lemon juice.
2. Season with salt and pepper and mix well.
3. Serve over a bed of mixed greens or with rice cakes.

Nutritional Facts (per serving):

- Calories: 250 | Protein: 30g | Carbs: 5g | Fat: 14g | Fiber: 2g

Substitution Variations:

- Use canned salmon instead of tuna for variety.
- Add avocado or capers for extra flavor.

Portion Control:

- One serving equals one can of tuna mixed with fresh vegetables, providing a lean protein meal.

Pro Tips:

- Pack this tuna salad in a mason jar for a portable, on-the-go lunch.
- Add a small handful of nuts or a piece of fruit for extra energy.

Baked Salmon with Steamed Asparagus

A nutrient-packed meal with omega-3 rich salmon and tender asparagus.

Estimated Meal Time: 20 minutes

Ingredients:

- 1 salmon fillet (4-6 oz)
- 1 bunch asparagus, trimmed
- 1 tbsp olive oil
- Salt and pepper to taste
- 1 lemon wedge

Cooking Method:

1. Preheat the oven to 400°F (200°C).
2. After putting the salmon fillet on a baking sheet, season it with salt and pepper and sprinkle it with olive oil.
3. Bake for 12-15 minutes, until the salmon is cooked through and flakes easily.
4. Steam the asparagus for 5-7 minutes until tender.
5. Serve the salmon with steamed asparagus and a squeeze of fresh lemon juice.

Nutritional Facts (per serving):

- Calories: 350 | Protein: 30g | Carbs: 8g | Fat: 24g | Fiber: 4g

Substitution Variations:

- Swap salmon for trout or cod.
- Add a side of quinoa or rice for extra carbs.

Portion Control:

- One serving includes 1 salmon fillet and a portion of asparagus.

Pro Tips:

- Use leftover salmon to top a salad or wrap in a gluten-free tortilla for another meal.
- For a richer flavor, top with a dollop of lactose-free sour cream or Greek yogurt.

Egg Salad on Gluten-Free Bread

A classic egg salad served on gluten-free bread for a hearty, gut-friendly lunch.

Estimated Meal Time: 15 minutes

Ingredients:

- 2 hard-boiled eggs, chopped
- 2 tbsp mayonnaise (low-FODMAP)
- 1 tsp Dijon mustard
- 1/4 cup chopped celery
- Salt and pepper to taste
- 2 slices gluten-free bread

Cooking Method:

1. In a bowl, combine the chopped eggs, mayonnaise, mustard, celery, salt, and pepper.
2. Spread the egg salad mixture on one slice of gluten-free bread.
3. Top with the second slice of bread, and serve immediately.

Nutritional Facts (per serving):

- Calories: 330 | Protein: 15g | Carbs: 18g | Fat: 24g | Fiber: 4g

Substitution Variations:

- Use plain Greek yogurt instead of mayonnaise for a lighter version.
- Add lettuce or tomato slices for extra freshness.

Portion Control:

- One serving equals one sandwich, providing a balanced lunch with protein and fiber.

Pro Tips:

- Make extra egg salad and store it in the fridge for a quick lunch the next day.
- Try using rice cakes instead of gluten-free bread for a lower-carb option.

Shrimp and Zucchini Stir-Fry with Rice

A quick stir-fry with shrimp and zucchini, served over rice for a light yet satisfying meal.

Estimated Meal Time: 15 minutes

Ingredients:

- 8 oz shrimp, peeled and deveined
- 1 medium zucchini, sliced
- 1 tbsp olive oil
- 1 tsp garlic-infused olive oil (low-FODMAP)
- 1/2 cup cooked white rice
- Salt and pepper to taste

Cooking Method:

1. Heat olive oil and garlic-infused oil in a skillet over medium heat.
2. Add the shrimp and cook for 3-4 minutes until pink and opaque.
3. Add the zucchini slices and cook for an additional 2-3 minutes until tender.
4. Serve the shrimp and zucchini stir-fry over the cooked rice.

Nutritional Facts (per serving):

- Calories: 280 | Protein: 28g | Carbs: 18g | Fat: 12g | Fiber: 3g

Substitution Variations:

- Swap shrimp for chicken or tofu for a different protein source.
- Add bell peppers or spinach for extra vegetables.

Portion Control:

- One serving includes 8 oz of shrimp and 1/2 cup of cooked rice.

Pro Tips:

- Make extra rice to use in other meals during the week.
- Use leftover stir-fry in wraps or salads for a quick meal.

Grilled Chicken and Avocado Salad

A refreshing salad with grilled chicken, creamy avocado, and a light dressing.

Estimated Meal Time: 20 minutes

Ingredients:

- 1 boneless, skinless chicken breast
- 1/2 avocado, sliced
- 4 cups mixed greens
- 1/4 cup cherry tomatoes, halved
- 1 tbsp olive oil
- 1 tbsp lemon juice
- Salt and pepper to taste

Cooking Method:

1. Grill the chicken breast for 6-7 minutes on each side until fully cooked.
2. Slice the chicken and place it on top of the mixed greens.
3. Add the sliced avocado, cherry tomatoes, and drizzle with olive oil and lemon juice.
4. Toss gently and serve.

Nutritional Facts (per serving):

- Calories: 350 | Protein: 30g | Carbs: 10g | Fat: 22g | Fiber: 6g

Substitution Variations:

- Swap chicken for grilled turkey or shrimp.
- Add a handful of nuts or seeds for added crunch.

Portion Control:

- One serving includes one chicken breast, a portion of salad, and avocado.

Pro Tips:

- Prepare extra grilled chicken for use in wraps, salads, or sandwiches throughout the week.
- Try a balsamic vinaigrette dressing for a tangy twist.

Low FODMAP Chicken Caesar Salad

A twist on the classic Caesar salad, made low FODMAP-friendly.

Estimated Meal Time: 20 minutes

Ingredients:

- 1 boneless, skinless chicken breast
- 4 cups romaine lettuce, chopped
- 1/4 cup lactose-free Parmesan cheese
- 1 tbsp olive oil
- 2 tbsp low-FODMAP Caesar dressing
- Salt and pepper to taste

Cooking Method:

1. Grill or cook the chicken breast until fully cooked, then slice it thinly.
2. In a large bowl, combine the romaine lettuce, Parmesan cheese, and sliced chicken.
3. Drizzle with low-FODMAP Caesar dressing and toss gently.
4. Serve immediately.

Nutritional Facts (per serving):

- Calories: 400 | Protein: 35g | Carbs: 12g | Fat: 24g | Fiber: 5g

Substitution Variations:

- Use grilled tofu or shrimp instead of chicken for a vegetarian or pescatarian option.
- Add gluten-free croutons for extra crunch.

Portion Control:

- One serving includes one chicken breast, a hearty portion of salad, and dressing.

Pro Tips:

- Make the salad ahead of time and pack the dressing separately to keep it fresh.

Quinoa and Cucumber Salad with Lemon Dressing

A refreshing, light salad made with quinoa, cucumber, and a zesty lemon dressing.

Estimated Meal Time: 15 minutes

Ingredients:

- 1 cup cooked quinoa
- 1 cucumber, diced
- 1/4 cup chopped fresh parsley
- 1 tbsp olive oil
- 1 tbsp lemon juice
- Salt and pepper to taste

Cooking Method:

1. In a large bowl, combine the cooked quinoa, diced cucumber, and parsley.
2. Season with salt and pepper and drizzle with lemon juice and olive oil.
3. Toss gently and serve.

Nutritional Facts (per serving):

- Calories: 220 | Protein: 6g | Carbs: 35g | Fat: 8g | Fiber: 4g

Substitution Variations:

- Add feta cheese or olives for extra flavor.
- Top with grilled chicken or shrimp for added protein.

Portion Control:

- One serving includes 1 cup of quinoa and a generous portion of vegetables.

Pro Tips:

- Prepare the quinoa salad in advance and refrigerate for a cool, refreshing lunch.
- For a spicier version, add a pinch of red pepper flakes to the dressing.

Grilled Vegetable and Hummus Wrap (using low FODMAP hummus)

A delicious, colorful wrap filled with grilled vegetables and creamy hummus, perfect for a light yet filling lunch.

Estimated Meal Time: 20 minutes

Ingredients:

- 1 whole wheat or gluten-free wrap (low FODMAP)
- 1/2 cup grilled mixed vegetables (zucchini, bell peppers, eggplant)
- 2 tbsp low-FODMAP hummus
- 1/4 cup spinach or arugula

Cooking Method:

1. Grill the mixed vegetables until soft and slightly charred.
2. Spread hummus on the wrap, then layer with grilled vegetables and spinach or arugula.
3. Roll up the wrap tightly and cut in half.
4. Serve immediately.

Nutritional Facts (per serving):

- Calories: 280 | Protein: 8g | Carbs: 30g | Fat: 15g | Fiber: 6g

Substitution Variations:

- Use a gluten-free wrap or lettuce leaves for a lower-carb version.
- Add grilled chicken or tofu for extra protein.

Portion Control:

- One serving equals one wrap.

Pro Tips:

- Wraps can be made ahead of time and stored in the fridge for a quick grab-and-go meal.
- Add avocado for extra creaminess and healthy fats.

Rice Paper Rolls with Shrimp and Vegetables

These fresh, colorful rice paper rolls are filled with shrimp and vegetables for a light and flavorful meal.

Estimated Meal Time: 20 minutes

Ingredients:

- 4 rice paper rolls
- 8-10 shrimp, cooked and peeled
- 1/2 cup shredded carrots
- 1/4 cup sliced cucumber
- Fresh cilantro or mint leaves
- 2 tbsp low-FODMAP dipping sauce (such as tamari or coconut aminos)

Cooking Method:

1. Soak rice paper rolls in warm water for 10-15 seconds until soft.
2. Layer the shrimp, shredded carrots, cucumber, and herbs on the rice paper.
3. Roll up the rice paper tightly, folding in the sides as you go.
4. Serve with dipping sauce.

Nutritional Facts (per serving):

- Calories: 150 | Protein: 15g | Carbs: 12g | Fat: 6g | Fiber: 2g

Substitution Variations:

- Use chicken or tofu for a different protein source.
- Add bell peppers or lettuce for extra crunch.

Portion Control:

- One serving consists of 4 rice paper rolls.

Pro Tips:

- Make extra rice paper rolls and refrigerate them for a quick snack.
- Customize the filling with your favorite low-FODMAP vegetables.

Turkey and Cucumber Rice Cakes

A simple, satisfying, and crunchy meal that's perfect for lunch or a snack.

Estimated Meal Time: 10 minutes

Ingredients:

- 2 plain rice cakes
- 4 slices deli turkey (ensure it's low-FODMAP)
- 1/2 cucumber, thinly sliced
- 1 tbsp mayonnaise (low-FODMAP)
- Salt and pepper to taste

Cooking Method:

1. Spread mayonnaise on the rice cakes.
2. Layer with slices of turkey and cucumber.
3. Sprinkle with salt and pepper, and serve.

Nutritional Facts (per serving):

- Calories: 230 | Protein: 16g | Carbs: 20g | Fat: 12g | Fiber: 3g

Substitution Variations:

- Use hummus or Greek yogurt in place of mayonnaise for a lighter version.
- Add lettuce or tomato for more veggies.

Portion Control:

- One serving equals 2 rice cakes topped with turkey and cucumber.

Pro Tips:

- Prepare rice cakes ahead of time for a quick meal during busy days.
- Use gluten-free rice cakes to keep the meal fully low FODMAP.

Baked Sweet Potato with Grilled Chicken

A nutritious and filling meal, combining the sweetness of baked sweet potatoes with protein-packed grilled chicken.

Estimated Meal Time: 30 minutes

Ingredients:

- 1 medium sweet potato
- 1 boneless, skinless chicken breast
- 1 tbsp olive oil
- Salt and pepper to taste
- 1 tsp smoked paprika (optional)

Cooking Method:

1. Preheat the oven to 400°F (200°C).
2. Wash and pierce the sweet potato with a fork. Bake for 25-30 minutes until soft.
3. While the sweet potato is baking, grill the chicken breast until fully cooked, about 6-7 minutes on each side.
4. Slice the sweet potato open and top with grilled chicken. Sprinkle with smoked paprika, if desired.
5. Serve immediately.

Nutritional Facts (per serving):

- Calories: 400 | Protein: 30g | Carbs: 45g | Fat: 15g | Fiber: 8g

Substitution Variations:

- Swap the chicken for turkey or tofu for a different protein.
- Add a drizzle of olive oil or your favorite low-FODMAP sauce on top.

Portion Control:

- One serving includes one baked sweet potato and one grilled chicken breast.

Pro Tips:

- Prepare extra grilled chicken for use in other meals throughout the week.

- Sweet potatoes can be baked in advance and reheated for a quick meal.

Chicken and Rice Soup with Carrots

A comforting and easy-to-digest soup with tender chicken, rice, and carrots.

Estimated Meal Time: 40 minutes

Ingredients:

- 2 boneless, skinless chicken breasts
- 1/2 cup cooked rice
- 2 large carrots, sliced
- 4 cups low-sodium chicken broth
- 1 tbsp olive oil
- Salt and pepper to taste

Cooking Method:

1. Heat olive oil in a large pot over medium heat. Cook until browned, about 6–7 minutes per side, after adding the chic ken breasts.
2. Remove the chicken and set aside. In the same pot, add the carrots and sauté for 3-4 minutes.
3. Add the chicken broth and bring to a simmer.
4. Return the chicken breasts to the pot and cook for an additional 15 minutes until fully cooked.
5. Shred the chicken and return it to the pot. Stir in the rice and season with salt and pepper.
6. Serve warm.

Nutritional Facts (per serving):

- Calories: 280 | Protein: 25g | Carbs: 30g | Fat: 8g | Fiber: 4g

Substitution Variations:

- Use turkey or tofu in place of chicken.
- Add other low-FODMAP vegetables like spinach or zucchini for more flavor.

Portion Control:

- One serving includes 1 cup of soup with chicken and rice.

Pro Tips:

- Make a big batch of this soup and store it in the fridge or freezer for later meals.
- Add fresh herbs like parsley for a burst of flavor.

Low FODMAP Chicken Tacos with Corn Tortillas

These delicious tacos are made with seasoned chicken and served on corn tortillas for a quick and satisfying lunch.

Estimated Meal Time: 20 minutes

Ingredients:

- 2 boneless, skinless chicken breasts, cooked and shredded
- 4 corn tortillas (ensure they are gluten-free and low-FODMAP)
- 1/2 cup shredded lettuce
- 1/4 cup diced tomatoes
- 1/4 cup lactose-free cheese (optional)
- 1 tbsp olive oil
- 1 tsp cumin
- Salt and pepper to taste

Cooking Method:

1. Shred the cooked chicken and toss it in olive oil, cumin, salt, and pepper.
2. Warm the corn tortillas in a skillet over medium heat for 1-2 minutes per side.
3. Assemble the tacos by adding seasoned chicken, lettuce, tomatoes, and cheese (if using).
4. Serve immediately.

Nutritional Facts (per serving):

- Calories: 350 | Protein: 30g | Carbs: 30g | Fat: 15g | Fiber: 6g

Substitution Variations:

- Use ground turkey or beef instead of chicken.
- Add avocado or a squeeze of lime for extra flavor.

Portion Control:

- One serving includes 2 tacos.

Pro Tips:

- Make the chicken ahead of time and store it for a quick taco night.
- Serve with a side of rice or grilled vegetables for a balanced meal.

FODMAP-Friendly Veggie Burger with Lettuce Wrap

A tasty, low FODMAP veggie burger that's light yet satisfying, served in place of a bun with crisp lettuce wraps.

Estimated Meal Time: 30 minutes

Ingredients:

- 1 can (15 oz) lentils, drained and rinsed
- 1/2 cup gluten-free breadcrumbs
- 1/4 cup grated zucchini (excess moisture squeezed out)
- 1 egg
- 1 tbsp garlic-infused oil (low FODMAP)
- 1/2 tsp cumin
- Salt and pepper to taste
- 4 large lettuce leaves (for wrapping)

Cooking Method:

1. In a mixing bowl, combine the lentils, breadcrumbs, grated zucchini, egg, garlic-infused oil, cumin, salt, and pepper.
2. Mash the mixture together until fully combined, then form into 4 patties.
3. Heat a non-stick skillet over medium heat, and cook the patties for 4-5 minutes per side, until golden and crispy.
4. Serve the patties on large lettuce leaves, wrapping them up as a bun alternative.

Nutritional Facts (per serving):

- Calories: 200 | Protein: 12g | Carbs: 25g | Fat: 8g | Fiber: 8g

Substitution Variations:

- Add some grated carrots or spinach to the veggie mixture for extra nutrients.
- Use chickpeas or black beans instead of lentils for a different texture.

Portion Control:

- One serving consists of one veggie burger wrapped in lettuce.

Pro Tips:

- Make extra patties and freeze them for future meals.
- Serve with a side of homemade low FODMAP fries for a complete meal.

Grilled Shrimp Skewers with Brown Rice

A light and protein-packed dish featuring succulent shrimp, paired with nutty brown rice.

Estimated Meal Time: 25 minutes

Ingredients:

- 10 large shrimp, peeled and deveined
- 1 tbsp olive oil
- 1 tsp paprika
- Salt and pepper to taste
- 1/2 cup cooked brown rice
- Lemon wedges for garnish

Cooking Method:

1. Preheat the grill or grill pan to medium heat.
2. Toss the shrimp in olive oil, paprika, salt, and pepper. Thread the shrimp onto skewers.
3. Grill the shrimp for 2-3 minutes on each side until pink and cooked through.
4. Serve the grilled shrimp over cooked brown rice and garnish with lemon wedges.

Nutritional Facts (per serving):

- Calories: 300 | Protein: 28g | Carbs: 30g | Fat: 10g | Fiber: 3g

Substitution Variations:

- Use chicken or tofu as an alternative to shrimp.
- Add steamed vegetables like broccoli or zucchini to the plate for more fiber.

Portion Control:

- One serving includes 10 shrimp and 1/2 cup of brown rice.

Pro Tips:

- Marinate the shrimp for 15-30 minutes before grilling for more flavor.

- Cook the rice ahead of time to save time during meal prep.

Cucumber and Tomato Salad with Olive Oil and Feta

A refreshing and vibrant salad, perfect for a light lunch or as a side dish.

Estimated Meal Time: 10 minutes

Ingredients:

- 1 cucumber, diced
- 1 cup cherry tomatoes, halved
- 1/4 cup feta cheese, crumbled
- 1 tbsp olive oil
- 1 tbsp lemon juice
- Salt and pepper to taste

Cooking Method:

1. In a bowl, combine the cucumber, cherry tomatoes, and feta cheese.
2. Drizzle with olive oil and lemon juice.
3. Season with salt and pepper, toss gently, and serve.

Nutritional Facts (per serving):

- Calories: 150 | Protein: 6g | Carbs: 12g | Fat: 12g | Fiber: 3g

Substitution Variations:

- Swap the feta for goat cheese or a dairy-free cheese alternative.
- Add fresh herbs like basil or parsley for extra flavor.

Portion Control:

- One serving includes about 1 cup of salad.

Pro Tips:

- Make extra dressing to use for other salads or vegetables throughout the week.
- Prepare the salad in advance but add the dressing just before serving to prevent wilting.

Beef Stir-Fry with Bell Peppers and Rice

A quick and flavorful stir-fry packed with tender beef, colorful bell peppers, and served with rice.

Estimated Meal Time: 20 minutes

Ingredients:

- 1 lb beef sirloin, thinly sliced
- 1 red bell pepper, thinly sliced
- 1 yellow bell pepper, thinly sliced
- 2 tbsp garlic-infused oil (low FODMAP)
- 1 tbsp soy sauce (low FODMAP)
- 1/2 cup cooked white rice
- Salt and pepper to taste

Cooking Method:

1. Heat the garlic-infused oil in a wok or large skillet over medium-high heat.
2. Add the beef and stir-fry for 3-4 minutes until browned.
3. Add the bell peppers and stir-fry for another 2-3 minutes until tender-crisp.
4. Add the soy sauce, salt, and pepper, and cook for another minute.
5. Serve the stir-fry over the cooked rice.

Nutritional Facts (per serving):

- Calories: 350 | Protein: 30g | Carbs: 35g | Fat: 12g | Fiber: 4g

Substitution Variations:

- Use chicken or tofu instead of beef.
- Add other low FODMAP vegetables like zucchini or spinach.

Portion Control:

- One serving includes 1/2 cup of rice and about 1 cup of stir-fry.

Pro Tips:

- Use pre-sliced beef or chicken to save time during preparation.
- Make extra stir-fry sauce and store it in the fridge for future meals.

These low FODMAP lunch recipes are not only gut-friendly but also full of flavor and nutrients. Whether you're in the mood for a light salad, a comforting stir-fry, or a satisfying veggie burger, these dishes will provide a variety of options to keep your lunch both delicious and healthy. Enjoy experimenting with these recipes and making them a regular part of your meal planning!

Dinner Recipes

Dinner is the perfect time to unwind and enjoy a satisfying, nutritious meal. These low FODMAP dinner recipes are designed to give you a hearty and flavorful meal that won't upset your digestive system. From grilled meats to veggie-packed dishes, these recipes are simple to prepare, full of flavor, and perfect for any night of the week.

Grilled Lemon Herb Chicken with Roasted Potatoes

A zesty, juicy chicken paired with crispy roasted potatoes—perfect for a filling and easy dinner.

Estimated Meal Time: 45 minutes

Ingredients:

- 2 boneless, skinless chicken breasts
- 1 tbsp garlic-infused oil (low FODMAP)
- 1 tbsp fresh lemon juice
- 1 tsp dried oregano
- Salt and pepper to taste
- 4 medium potatoes, cut into wedges

Cooking Method:

1. Preheat the oven to 400°F (200°C).
2. In a small bowl, mix garlic-infused oil, lemon juice, oregano, salt, and pepper.
3. Rub the chicken breasts with the lemon herb mixture.
4. Arrange the potato wedges on a baking sheet and drizzle with olive oil, salt, and pepper. Roast for 30-35 minutes, flipping halfway.
5. Grill the chicken on medium-high heat for 5-7 minutes per side until cooked through.
6. Serve the grilled chicken alongside the roasted potatoes.

Nutritional Facts (per serving):

- Calories: 400 | Protein: 35g | Carbs: 45g | Fat: 12g | Fiber: 7g

Substitution Variations:

- Swap chicken for turkey breasts for a leaner option.
- Add herbs like thyme or rosemary for added flavor.

Portion Control:

- One serving consists of one chicken breast and about 1 cup of roasted potatoes.

Pro Tips:

- Prepare the potatoes in advance and store them in the fridge until ready to bake.
- For extra flavor, marinate the chicken for a few hours before grilling.

Baked Cod with Roasted Carrots and Green Beans

A light, healthy dinner that's full of flavor and easy to prepare.

Estimated Meal Time: 30 minutes

Ingredients:

- 2 cod fillets
- 1 tbsp olive oil
- Salt and pepper to taste
- 1 cup carrots, sliced
- 1 cup green beans, trimmed
- 1 tsp fresh parsley, chopped

Cooking Method:

1. Preheat the oven to 375°F (190°C).
2. Place the cod fillets on a baking sheet, drizzle with olive oil, and season with salt and pepper.
3. On a separate baking sheet, arrange the carrots and green beans, drizzle with olive oil, and season.
4. Bake the cod for 15-18 minutes, or until it flakes easily with a fork.
5. Roast the vegetables for 20-25 minutes, stirring halfway through.

6. Serve the cod with the roasted vegetables, garnished with parsley.

Nutritional Facts (per serving):

- Calories: 300 | Protein: 30g | Carbs: 25g | Fat: 12g | Fiber: 6g

Substitution Variations:

- Substitute cod for tilapia or haddock.
- Try adding roasted sweet potatoes instead of carrots for variety.

Portion Control:

- One serving includes 1 cod fillet and 1 cup of vegetables.

Pro Tips:

- Use a meat thermometer to check the cod's doneness (145°F or 63°C).
- Roast the vegetables in advance to save time during the week.

Beef and Vegetable Stir-Fry with Rice

A quick, colorful stir-fry that's loaded with vegetables and protein-packed beef.

Estimated Meal Time: 20 minutes

Ingredients:

- 1 lb lean beef, thinly sliced
- 1 cup bell peppers, sliced
- 1/2 cup carrots, julienned
- 1/2 cup snap peas
- 1 tbsp garlic-infused oil (low FODMAP)
- 2 tbsp soy sauce (low FODMAP)
- 1 tbsp sesame oil
- 1 cup cooked rice

Cooking Method:

1. Heat garlic-infused oil in a large skillet over medium-high heat.
2. Add the sliced beef and stir-fry for 3-4 minutes until browned.
3. Add the bell peppers, carrots, and snap peas, stir-fry for an additional 3-4 minutes.
4. Add soy sauce and sesame oil, stir to coat everything.
5. Serve the stir-fry over a bed of cooked rice.

Nutritional Facts (per serving):

- Calories: 350 | Protein: 32g | Carbs: 40g | Fat: 12g | Fiber: 5g

Substitution Variations:

- Use chicken or tofu in place of beef.
- Switch to quinoa instead of rice for added protein.

Portion Control:

- One serving includes 1 cup of stir-fry and 1/2 cup of rice.

Pro Tips:

- Make extra stir-fry and store it in the fridge for lunch the next day.
- Use pre-sliced vegetables to save time.

Low FODMAP Chicken Alfredo with Zucchini Noodles

A creamy, satisfying dish without the heaviness of traditional pasta—perfect for a low FODMAP lifestyle.

Estimated Meal Time: 25 minutes

Ingredients:

- 2 chicken breasts, grilled and sliced
- 2 medium zucchinis, spiralized into noodles
- 1/2 cup lactose-free cream
- 1/4 cup grated Parmesan cheese
- 1 tbsp garlic-infused oil (low FODMAP)
- Salt and pepper to taste

Cooking Method:

1. Heat garlic-infused oil in a pan over medium heat.
2. Add the zucchini noodles and sauté for 2-3 minutes until tender but not mushy.
3. In a separate saucepan, heat the lactose-free cream and stir in the Parmesan until smooth and creamy.
4. Add the grilled chicken to the sauce and simmer for 2 minutes.
5. Toss the zucchini noodles with the chicken Alfredo sauce and serve.

Nutritional Facts (per serving):

- Calories: 350 | Protein: 35g | Carbs: 15g | Fat: 18g | Fiber: 4g

Substitution Variations:

- Use gluten-free pasta if you prefer a traditional noodle option.
- Replace chicken with shrimp for a different protein.

Portion Control:

- One serving includes about 1 cup of zucchini noodles with 1/2 chicken breast and sauce.

Pro Tips:

- Use a spiralizer for perfectly shaped zucchini noodles.

- Prepare the sauce in advance to make the meal quicker on busy nights.

- Use a spiralizer for perfectly shaped zucchini noodles.

Grilled Salmon with Steamed Broccoli

A light and healthy dinner option featuring omega-3-rich salmon and nutrient-packed broccoli.

Estimated Meal Time: 20 minutes

Ingredients:

- 2 salmon fillets
- 1 tbsp olive oil
- 1 lemon, sliced
- 2 cups broccoli florets
- Salt and pepper to taste

Cooking Method:

1. Preheat the grill to medium-high heat.
2. Rub the salmon fillets with olive oil, salt, and pepper, and place lemon slices on top.
3. Grill the salmon for 4-5 minutes per side until fully cooked.
4. Steam the broccoli florets for 4-5 minutes until tender.
5. Serve the grilled salmon with the steamed broccoli.

Nutritional Facts (per serving):

- Calories: 400 | Protein: 35g | Carbs: 15g | Fat: 25g | Fiber: 5g

Substitution Variations:

- Substitute salmon with another fatty fish like trout or mackerel.
- Add other steamed vegetables, such as asparagus or green beans, to the plate.

Portion Control:

- One serving consists of one salmon fillet and about 1 cup of steamed broccoli.

Pro Tips:

- Marinate the salmon in a lemon and herb mix for extra flavor.
- Cook the broccoli in a steamer basket for perfect texture without overcooking.

Stuffed Bell Peppers with Ground Turkey and Quinoa

A satisfying, healthy dinner that's full of flavor, fiber, and protein.

Estimated Meal Time: 40 minutes

Ingredients:

- 4 large bell peppers, tops cut off and seeds removed
- 1 lb ground turkey
- 1 cup cooked quinoa
- 1 tsp garlic-infused oil (low FODMAP)
- 1/2 cup diced tomatoes (canned or fresh, no added garlic or onion)
- 1/2 cup shredded cheese (optional)
- Salt and pepper to taste

Cooking Method:

1. Preheat the oven to 375°F (190°C).
2. Heat garlic-infused oil in a skillet over medium heat. Add the ground turkey and cook until browned, about 5-7 minutes.
3. Stir in the cooked quinoa, diced tomatoes, salt, and pepper. Cook for another 2-3 minutes, then remove from heat.
4. Stuff the bell peppers with the turkey and quinoa mixture, pressing the filling firmly inside.
5. Place the stuffed peppers in a baking dish and bake for 25-30 minutes. If using cheese, sprinkle on top and bake for an additional 5 minutes until melted.
6. Serve hot.

Nutritional Facts (per serving):

- Calories: 350 | Protein: 30g | Carbs: 30g | Fat: 12g | Fiber: 7g

Substitution Variations:

- Swap turkey for ground chicken or beef.

- Use brown rice instead of quinoa if preferred.

Portion Control:

- One stuffed pepper is a complete serving.

Pro Tips:

- Make extra filling and store for a quick meal later in the week.
- Add some chopped spinach or zucchini to the filling for extra veggies.

Baked Chicken Thighs with Sweet Potato Wedges

A hearty and comforting dinner that's simple to make and perfect for busy nights.

Estimated Meal Time: 45 minutes

Ingredients:

- 4 bone-in, skin-on chicken thighs
- 2 large sweet potatoes, cut into wedges
- 1 tbsp garlic-infused oil (low FODMAP)
- 1 tbsp olive oil
- 1 tsp paprika
- Salt and pepper to taste
- 1/2 tsp dried rosemary

Cooking Method:

1. Preheat the oven to 400°F (200°C).
2. Combine the sweet potato wedges, paprika, rosemary, salt, pepper, and oil flavored with garlic in a bowl.
3. Place the sweet potatoes on a baking sheet and bake for 20 minutes.
4. Rub the chicken thighs with olive oil, salt, and pepper.
5. After 20 minutes, add the chicken thighs to the baking sheet with the sweet potatoes.
   The internal temperature of the chicken should reach 165°F (74°C) after another 25 to 30 minutes of baking.
6. Serve the baked chicken thighs with the roasted sweet potatoes.

Nutritional Facts (per serving):

- Calories: 400 | Protein: 30g | Carbs: 35g | Fat: 20g | Fiber: 6g

Substitution Variations:

- Use chicken breasts if you prefer leaner meat.
- Add some roasted Brussels sprouts to the tray for an extra vegetable.

Portion Control:

- One serving consists of one chicken thigh and 1 cup of sweet potato wedges.

Pro Tips:

- Use parchment paper to prevent sticking and make clean-up easier.
- For extra crispiness, broil the chicken for the last 2-3 minutes.

Shrimp and Spinach Stir-Fry with Rice Noodles

A light and flavorful stir-fry that's packed with protein and healthy vegetables.

Estimated Meal Time: 20 minutes

Ingredients:

- 1 lb shrimp, peeled and deveined
- 2 cups fresh spinach, roughly chopped
- 1 cup rice noodles, cooked
- 1 tbsp garlic-infused oil (low FODMAP)
- 1 tbsp soy sauce (low FODMAP)
- 1 tbsp sesame oil
- 1/2 tsp ginger, grated
- 1/4 tsp red pepper flakes (optional)

Cooking Method:

1. Heat garlic-infused oil in a large skillet over medium-high heat.
2. Add the shrimp and cook for 2-3 minutes per side until pink and cooked through. Remove from the skillet.
3. In the same skillet, add the spinach and cook for 1-2 minutes until wilted.
4. Stir in the cooked rice noodles, soy sauce, sesame oil, ginger, and red pepper flakes (if using). Cook for another 2-3 minutes, then return the shrimp to the skillet.
5. Toss everything together and serve hot.

Nutritional Facts (per serving):

- Calories: 350 | Protein: 30g | Carbs: 35g | Fat: 12g | Fiber: 4g

Substitution Variations:

- Replace shrimp with chicken or tofu for a different protein.

- Add other low FODMAP veggies, such as bell peppers or zucchini.

Portion Control:

- One serving includes 1 cup of stir-fry and 1/2 cup of rice noodles.

Pro Tips:

- Use a wok or large skillet for better heat distribution.

- Make extra rice noodles to use in salads or other stir-fries.

Pan-Seared Steak with Mashed Potatoes and Green Beans

A satisfying dinner with tender steak and creamy mashed potatoes.

Estimated Meal Time: 30 minutes

Ingredients:

- 2 steaks (such as ribeye or sirloin)
- 4 medium potatoes, peeled and cubed
- 1 tbsp garlic-infused oil (low FODMAP)
- 1 cup green beans, trimmed
- 1/4 cup lactose-free butter
- Salt and pepper to taste

Cooking Method:

1. Boil the potatoes in salted water until tender, about 15-20 minutes. Drain and mash with lactose-free butter and salt.
2. While the potatoes are cooking, heat garlic-infused oil in a skillet over medium-high heat.
3. Season the steaks with salt and pepper, then pan-sear for 4-5 minutes per side, depending on thickness, until cooked to your desired doneness.
4. Steam the green beans for 5-7 minutes until tender.
5. Serve the pan-seared steak with mashed potatoes and green beans.

Nutritional Facts (per serving):

- Calories: 500 | Protein: 40g | Carbs: 40g | Fat: 22g | Fiber: 6g

Substitution Variations:

- Substitute the steak for grilled chicken or pork chops.
- Swap green beans for another low FODMAP vegetable like carrots or zucchini.

Portion Control:

- One serving consists of one steak, 1/2 cup of mashed potatoes, and 1 cup of green beans.

Pro Tips:

- Let the steak rest for 5 minutes before slicing to retain juices.
- Use a potato ricer for extra smooth mashed potatoes.

Chicken and Rice Casserole with Low FODMAP Veggies

A one-pan, comforting casserole that's easy to make and full of flavor.

Estimated Meal Time: 45 minutes

Ingredients:

- 2 chicken breasts, cooked and shredded
- 1 cup cooked rice
- 1/2 cup lactose-free cream
- 1/2 cup shredded cheese (optional)
- 1 cup low FODMAP veggies (e.g., carrots, spinach, zucchini)
- Salt and pepper to taste

Cooking Method:

1. Preheat the oven to 375°F (190°C).
2. In a large bowl, combine the shredded chicken, cooked rice, low FODMAP veggies, lactose-free cream, salt, and pepper.
3. Pour the mixture into a greased casserole dish and sprinkle with shredded cheese if desired.
4. Bake for 25-30 minutes, until the casserole is hot and bubbly.
5. Serve warm.

Nutritional Facts (per serving):

- Calories: 400 | Protein: 35g | Carbs: 40g | Fat: 15g | Fiber: 6g

Substitution Variations:

- Use quinoa instead of rice for a higher-protein option.
- Add a handful of fresh herbs like thyme or parsley for more flavor.

Portion Control:

- One serving consists of 1 cup of casserole.

Pro Tips:

- Prepare the casserole in advance and refrigerate for a quick meal later.
- For extra crunch, top with gluten-free breadcrumbs before baking.

Grilled Vegetable Skewers with Quinoa

These vibrant and flavorful grilled vegetable skewers are paired with quinoa, making for a hearty yet light dinner option. Perfect for a summer evening or a quick meal anytime.

Estimated Meal Time: 30 minutes

Ingredients:

- 1 red bell pepper, cut into chunks
- 1 zucchini, sliced
- 1 red onion, cut into chunks
- 1 cup cherry tomatoes
- 1 cup quinoa, cooked
- 2 tbsp olive oil
- 1 tsp dried oregano
- Salt and pepper to taste
- Fresh parsley for garnish (optional)

Cooking Method:

1. Preheat the grill to medium-high heat.
2. Alternately thread different kinds and colors of veggies onto skewers.
3. Drizzle the vegetables with olive oil, oregano, salt, and pepper.
4. Grill the vegetable skewers for 8-10 minutes, turning occasionally, until they are charred and tender.
5. While grilling, cook the quinoa according to package instructions.
6. Serve the grilled vegetables on a bed of quinoa, garnished with fresh parsley if desired.

Nutritional Facts (per serving):

- Calories: 250 | Protein: 7g | Carbs: 35g | Fat: 12g | Fiber: 6g

Substitution Variations:

- Swap in your favorite veggies such as eggplant, mushrooms, or squash.
- Use brown rice or couscous instead of quinoa for variety.

Portion Control:

- One serving includes 2-3 skewers and 1/2 cup of quinoa.

Pro Tips:

- For added flavor, marinate the vegetables in olive oil and herbs for 30 minutes before grilling.
- If you don't have a grill, roast the vegetables in the oven at 400°F (200°C) for 15-20 minutes.

Zucchini Lasagna with Ground Turkey

A healthier twist on classic lasagna, this zucchini-based version uses thin slices of zucchini instead of pasta, making it a light yet filling option for dinner.

Estimated Meal Time: 40 minutes

Ingredients:

- 3 medium zucchinis, sliced thinly lengthwise
- 1 lb ground turkey
- 1 1/2 cups low-sodium tomato sauce (no added garlic or onion)
- 1 cup ricotta cheese (lactose-free if needed)
- 1 cup shredded mozzarella cheese (lactose-free if needed)
- 1/2 tsp dried basil
- Salt and pepper to taste
- Olive oil for greasing

Cooking Method:

1. Preheat the oven to 375°F (190°C).
2. Lightly grease a baking dish with olive oil.
3. In a skillet, cook the ground turkey until browned, then stir in the tomato sauce, basil, salt, and pepper. Simmer for 5 minutes.
4. Layer the zucchini slices at the bottom of the baking dish. Spread a layer of turkey sauce, followed by a layer of ricotta

cheese. Repeat the layers until all ingredients are used.

5. Top with mozzarella cheese and bake for 25-30 minutes, until bubbly and golden.
6. Let it rest for 5 minutes before serving.

Nutritional Facts (per serving):

- Calories: 350 | Protein: 30g | Carbs: 15g | Fat: 20g | Fiber: 4g

Substitution Variations:

- You can use ground chicken or beef instead of turkey.

- Try using dairy-free cheese for a completely lactose-free version.

Portion Control:

- One serving includes a generous 1-cup portion of lasagna.

Pro Tips:

- Use a mandoline slicer for perfectly even zucchini slices.
- To reduce moisture, salt the zucchini slices and let them sit for 15 minutes before layering.

Baked Lemon Garlic Salmon with Roasted Asparagus

A simple, nutrient-packed dinner that is easy to prepare and full of flavor, this salmon is baked with lemon and garlic, then served alongside roasted asparagus.

Estimated Meal Time: 30 minutes

Ingredients:

- 2 salmon fillets
- 1 lemon, sliced
- 2 cloves garlic, minced (or garlic-infused oil for low FODMAP)
- 1 tbsp olive oil
- 1 bunch asparagus, trimmed
- Salt and pepper to taste

Cooking Method:

1. Preheat the oven to 400°F (200°C).
2. Arrange the salmon fillets on a parchment paper-lined baking pan.
3. Drizzle with olive oil, and season with salt, pepper, minced garlic (or garlic-infused oil), and lemon slices.
4. Arrange the asparagus on the same baking sheet and drizzle with olive oil. Season with salt and pepper.
5. Bake for 15-20 minutes, or until the salmon is cooked through and flakes easily with a fork, and the asparagus is tender.
6. Serve the salmon with roasted asparagus on the side.

Nutritional Facts (per serving):

- Calories: 400 | Protein: 35g | Carbs: 10g | Fat: 25g | Fiber: 5g

Substitution Variations:

- Swap salmon for any other fish, such as trout or tilapia.
- If you prefer, you can substitute broccoli or green beans for asparagus.

Portion Control:

- One serving includes 1 salmon fillet and 1/2 cup of roasted asparagus.

Pro Tips:

- For a zesty twist, drizzle the baked salmon with fresh lemon juice right before serving.
- If you prefer your asparagus extra crispy, roast it for an additional 5-10 minutes.

Low FODMAP Beef Tacos with Corn Tortillas

These beef tacos are a satisfying and easy dinner, made with ground beef and topped with fresh veggies, all wrapped in a gluten-free corn tortilla.

Estimated Meal Time: 30 minutes

Ingredients:

- 1 lb ground beef
- 1 tsp cumin
- 1 tsp chili powder
- Salt and pepper to taste
- 8 small corn tortillas
- 1/2 cup shredded lettuce
- 1/4 cup diced tomatoes
- 1/4 cup shredded cheddar cheese (optional)
- 1/4 cup avocado slices

Cooking Method:

1. In a skillet, cook the ground beef over medium heat until browned.
2. Add the cumin, chili powder, salt, and pepper to the beef, stirring to combine. Cook for another 3-4 minutes.
3. Warm the corn tortillas in a dry skillet or microwave.
4. Assemble the tacos by filling each tortilla with the seasoned beef, shredded lettuce, diced tomatoes, shredded cheese (if using), and avocado slices.
5. Serve immediately.

Nutritional Facts (per serving):

- Calories: 350 | Protein: 25g | Carbs: 30g | Fat: 18g | Fiber: 5g

Substitution Variations:

- Use ground turkey or chicken instead of beef for a leaner option.

- Add sautéed bell peppers or onions (if tolerated) for extra flavor.

Portion Control:

- One serving includes 2 tacos.

Pro Tips:

- To reduce the fat content, drain the fat from the beef after browning.

- Warm the tortillas before assembling the tacos to make them more pliable.

Grilled Chicken with Sweet Potato Fries

A simple yet delicious dinner featuring tender grilled chicken paired with crispy sweet potato fries for a satisfying, healthy meal.

Estimated Meal Time: 40 minutes

Ingredients:

- 2 boneless, skinless chicken breasts
- 2 medium sweet potatoes, cut into fries
- 1 tbsp olive oil
- 1 tsp paprika
- Salt and pepper to taste
- 1 tbsp garlic-infused oil (optional for seasoning)

Cooking Method:

1. Preheat the oven to 425°F (220°C).
2. Toss the sweet potato fries with olive oil, paprika, salt, and pepper. Arrange them on a baking sheet in a single layer.
3. Bake for 25-30 minutes, flipping halfway through, until the fries are crispy and golden.
4. Meanwhile, grill the chicken breasts on medium heat for 6-8 minutes per side, until cooked through.
5. Serve the grilled chicken with sweet potato fries on the side.

Nutritional Facts (per serving):

- Calories: 450 | Protein: 35g | Carbs: 45g | Fat: 15g | Fiber: 7g

Substitution Variations:

- Use any favorite spices, such as cumin or rosemary, for the sweet potato fries.
- Try grilled salmon or turkey burgers in place of chicken.

Portion Control:

- One serving includes 1 chicken breast and 1 cup of sweet potato fries.

Pro Tips:

- For extra crispy fries, soak the sweet potato slices in water for 30 minutes before baking.
- Season the chicken with fresh herbs like thyme or rosemary for added flavor.

Chicken and Spinach Stuffed Portobello Mushrooms

These hearty portobello mushrooms are stuffed with a delicious mixture of chicken and spinach, creating a satisfying and flavorful meal that's easy to prepare.

Estimated Meal Time: 35 minutes

Ingredients:

- 4 large portobello mushrooms, stems removed
- 1 lb ground chicken
- 2 cups fresh spinach, chopped
- 1/2 cup ricotta cheese (lactose-free if needed)
- 1/4 cup grated Parmesan cheese
- 1 tsp garlic-infused oil
- Salt and pepper to taste
- Olive oil for greasing

Cooking Method:

1. Preheat the oven to 375°F (190°C).
2. Lightly grease a baking sheet with olive oil.
3. In a skillet, heat the garlic-infused oil and cook the ground chicken over medium heat until browned and fully cooked.
4. Stir in the chopped spinach and cook until wilted. Remove from heat and mix in the ricotta and Parmesan cheeses. Season with salt and pepper.
5. Stuff the portobello mushroom caps with the chicken-spinach mixture and place them on the prepared baking sheet.
6. Bake for 20-25 minutes until the mushrooms are tender and the filling is hot.

Nutritional Facts (per serving):

- Calories: 350 | Protein: 35g | Carbs: 10g |
  Fat: 20g | Fiber: 4g

Substitution Variations:

- Use ground turkey or lean beef for a
  different flavor.
- Replace ricotta with cottage cheese for a
  slightly different texture.

Portion Control:

- One serving consists of 1 stuffed
  portobello mushroom.

Pro Tips:

- Make sure to remove the mushroom
  stems thoroughly to create more room for
  the filling.
- You can grill the mushrooms instead of
  baking for a smoky flavor.

Shrimp and Cucumber Salad with Lemon Dressing

This light and refreshing salad combine succulent shrimp with crisp cucumber, tossed in a zesty lemon dressing, perfect for a quick and healthy dinner.

Estimated Meal Time: 20 minutes

Ingredients:

- 1 lb shrimp, peeled and deveined
- 1 cucumber, thinly sliced
- 1/4 red onion, thinly sliced (optional, if tolerated)
- 1 tbsp fresh dill, chopped
- 2 tbsp olive oil
- 2 tbsp fresh lemon juice
- 1 tsp Dijon mustard
- Salt and pepper to taste

Cooking Method:

1. In a skillet, cook the shrimp over medium heat for 2-3 minutes per side until pink and cooked through. Remove from heat and let them cool.
2. In a large bowl, combine the cucumber, red onion (if using), and dill.
3. In a small bowl, whisk together the olive oil, lemon juice, Dijon mustard, salt, and pepper to create the dressing.
4. Toss the cooked shrimp with the cucumber mixture and drizzle with the lemon dressing.
5. Serve immediately or chill for 10-15 minutes to let the flavors meld.

Nutritional Facts (per serving):

- Calories: 250 | Protein: 28g | Carbs: 8g | Fat: 14g | Fiber: 2g

Substitution Variations:

- Use grilled chicken or scallops instead of shrimp.

- Add avocado slices for extra creaminess.

Portion Control:

- One serving is about 1 cup of salad with 4-5 shrimp.

Pro Tips:

- To add crunch, toss in some chopped nuts like almonds or walnuts.
- Make the salad ahead of time and refrigerate for a quick dinner or lunch.

Low FODMAP Meatballs with Rice and Marinara Sauce

These tender meatballs are made with ground beef and served with a rich marinara sauce and fluffy rice, providing a comforting and filling dinner.

Estimated Meal Time: 45 minutes

Ingredients:

- 1 lb ground beef
- 1/2 cup gluten-free breadcrumbs
- 1 egg
- 1 tsp dried oregano
- 1/2 tsp garlic-infused oil
- 2 cups low-sodium marinara sauce (no garlic or onion)
- 1 cup white rice, cooked
- Salt and pepper to taste

Cooking Method:

1. Preheat the oven to 375°F (190°C).
2. In a large bowl, combine the ground beef, breadcrumbs, egg, oregano, garlic-infused oil, salt, and pepper. Mix until well combined and form into 12 meatballs.
3. Arrange the meatballs on a baking sheet lined with parchment paper and bake for 20-25 minutes, until browned and cooked through.
4. While the meatballs are baking, heat the marinara sauce in a saucepan over low heat.
5. Serve the meatballs over cooked rice and top with marinara sauce.

Nutritional Facts (per serving):

- Calories: 350 | Protein: 30g | Carbs: 25g | Fat: 18g | Fiber: 3g

Substitution Variations:

- Use ground turkey or chicken for a lighter version of the meatballs.
- Serve the meatballs with quinoa or mashed sweet potatoes instead of rice.

Portion Control:

- One serving includes 3 meatballs and 1/2 cup of rice.

Pro Tips:

- For extra flavor, add chopped fresh parsley to the meatball mixture.
- Make the meatballs in advance and freeze them for easy future meals.

Grilled Chicken with Roasted Brussels Sprouts

This simple yet flavorful dinner features grilled chicken paired with roasted Brussels sprouts for a delicious, nutrient-packed meal.

Estimated Meal Time: 35 minutes

Ingredients:

- 2 boneless, skinless chicken breasts
- 1 lb Brussels sprouts, halved
- 2 tbsp olive oil
- 1 tsp dried thyme
- Salt and pepper to taste
- 1 lemon, sliced (optional)

Cooking Method:

1. Preheat the grill to medium heat.
2. Season the chicken breasts with olive oil, salt, pepper, and dried thyme. Grill for 6-8 minutes per side, or until fully cooked.
3. While the chicken is grilling, preheat the oven to 400°F (200°C).
4. Toss the halved Brussels sprouts with olive oil, salt, pepper, and thyme. Spread them out in a single layer on a baking sheet.
5. Roast for 20-25 minutes, flipping halfway through, until crispy and tender.
6. Serve the grilled chicken with roasted Brussels sprouts and lemon slices on the side.

Nutritional Facts (per serving):

- Calories: 400 | Protein: 35g | Carbs: 18g | Fat: 22g | Fiber: 7g

Substitution Variations:

- Replace Brussels sprouts with other low FODMAP veggies like zucchini or green beans.
- Add a side of mashed potatoes for a heartier meal.

Portion Control:

- One serving includes 1 chicken breast and 1 cup of Brussels sprouts.

Pro Tips:

- If you prefer softer Brussels sprouts, cover them with foil during the first 10 minutes of roasting.
- For added flavor, drizzle the Brussels sprouts with balsamic vinegar before serving.

Baked Eggplant with Ground Beef and Mozzarella

This low FODMAP-friendly baked eggplant is topped with a savory ground beef mixture and melted mozzarella for a delicious, filling dinner.

Estimated Meal Time: 40 minutes

Ingredients:

- 2 medium eggplants, sliced into 1/2-inch rounds
- 1 lb ground beef
- 1 cup mozzarella cheese, shredded (lactose-free if needed)
- 1/2 cup tomato sauce (low FODMAP)
- 1 tsp dried basil
- Salt and pepper to taste
- Olive oil for greasing

Cooking Method:

1. Preheat the oven to 375°F (190°C).
2. Lightly grease a baking dish with olive oil and arrange the eggplant slices in a single layer.
3. In a skillet, cook the ground beef over medium heat until browned. Add the tomato sauce, basil, salt, and pepper, and simmer for 5 minutes.
4. Spoon the beef mixture over each eggplant slice and top with shredded mozzarella.
5. Bake for 20-25 minutes, or until the cheese is melted and bubbly.

Nutritional Facts (per serving):

- Calories: 350 | Protein: 30g | Carbs: 12g | Fat: 22g | Fiber: 5g

Substitution Variations:

- Swap ground beef with ground turkey or chicken for a leaner option.

- Use dairy-free cheese to make this recipe fully dairy-free.

Portion Control:

- One serving includes 3-4 eggplant slices with ground beef and cheese.

Pro Tips:

- To reduce bitterness, sprinkle the eggplant slices with salt and let them sit for 15 minutes before cooking.

- For extra flavor, top with fresh basil before serving.

These Low FODMAP dinner recipes are easy to prepare and provide satisfying, nutritious meals that support your digestive health. Whether you're craving something light like grilled salmon or hearty like stuffed bell peppers, there's a dish to suit every taste. Enjoy your delicious, gut-friendly meals while maintaining a balanced lifestyle!

Snack Recipes

Sometimes, you just need a quick, satisfying snack to keep you going through the day. These low FODMAP-friendly snacks are perfect for when hunger strikes between meals. They're simple to prepare, full of flavor, and gentle on your digestive system. Whether you're craving something crunchy, creamy, or a bit of sweetness, you'll find the perfect option here.

Rice Cakes with Peanut Butter and Strawberries

This easy snack combines the crunch of rice cakes with the creamy richness of peanut butter and the natural sweetness of fresh strawberries.

Estimated Meal Time: 5 minutes

Ingredients:

- 2 rice cakes
- 2 tbsp peanut butter (check for added sugars and low FODMAP)
- 4-5 fresh strawberries, sliced
- A drizzle of honey (optional)

Cooking Method:

1. Spread the peanut butter evenly over each rice cake.
2. Top with sliced strawberries.
3. Drizzle with honey if you like a touch of extra sweetness.

Nutritional Facts (per serving):

- Calories: 250 | Protein: 6g | Carbs: 24g | Fat: 16g | Fiber: 4g

Substitution Variations:

- Swap peanut butter for almond butter if preferred.
- Use other fruits like blueberries or raspberries if strawberries aren't available.

Portion Control:

- One serving consists of 2 rice cakes topped with peanut butter and strawberries.

Pro Tips:

- For added crunch, try using whole grain rice cakes.
- Make this snack even more satisfying by adding a sprinkle of chia seeds for extra fiber.

Carrot and Cucumber Sticks with Low FODMAP Hummus

A crunchy and refreshing snack, this combination of carrot and cucumber sticks paired with low FODMAP hummus is both nutritious and satisfying.

Estimated Meal Time: 5 minutes

Ingredients:

- 1 medium carrot, peeled and cut into sticks
- 1/2 cucumber, sliced into sticks
- 1/4 cup low FODMAP hummus

Cooking Method:

1. Peel and cut the carrot into sticks and slice the cucumber into thin strips.
2. Serve with a side of low FODMAP hummus for dipping.

Nutritional Facts (per serving):

- Calories: 120 | Protein: 4g | Carbs: 15g | Fat: 7g | Fiber: 5g

Substitution Variations:

- Swap the hummus for a yogurt-based dip if you prefer a lighter option.
- Add a sprinkle of herbs like parsley or dill to the hummus for extra flavor.

Portion Control:

- One serving is about 1/2 cup of vegetables with 1/4 cup hummus.

Pro Tips:

- Store pre-cut veggies in the fridge for a quick grab-and-go snack.

- You can use other low FODMAP vegetables such as bell peppers or zucchini.

Almonds and Walnuts Snack Mix

This easy snack mix is a perfect blend of crunchy almonds and walnuts, providing healthy fats and protein to keep you satisfied.

Estimated Meal Time: 3 minutes

Ingredients:

- 1/4 cup almonds
- 1/4 cup walnuts
- A pinch of sea salt (optional)

Cooking Method:

1. Combine the almonds and walnuts in a small bowl.
2. Toss with a pinch of sea salt if desired.

Nutritional Facts (per serving):

- Calories: 200 | Protein: 6g | Carbs: 6g | Fat: 18g | Fiber: 3g

Substitution Variations:

- Add pumpkin seeds or sunflower seeds for extra crunch.
- Swap out walnuts for pecans if preferred.

Portion Control:

- One serving is approximately 1/2 cup of mixed nuts.

Pro Tips:

- Pre-portion this snack into small containers for easy, on-the-go options.
- Roasting the nuts lightly can enhance the flavor.

Low FODMAP Popcorn with Olive Oil and Sea Salt

Popcorn is a great low FODMAP snack, and when prepared with olive oil and sea salt, it's a healthy, flavorful option.

Estimated Meal Time: 10 minutes

Ingredients:

- 1/4 cup popcorn kernels
- 1 tbsp olive oil
- A pinch of sea salt

Cooking Method:

1. Heat a large pot over medium heat and add the olive oil.
2. Add the popcorn kernels and cover the pot. Shake occasionally to ensure even popping.
3. Once popped, sprinkle with sea salt and serve.

Nutritional Facts (per serving):

- Calories: 150 | Protein: 3g | Carbs: 20g | Fat: 7g | Fiber: 3g

Substitution Variations:

- Add a sprinkle of grated Parmesan or a dash of paprika for a different flavor.
- Use melted butter instead of olive oil for a richer taste.

Portion Control:

- One serving is about 3 cups of popped popcorn.

Pro Tips:

- Store popped popcorn in an airtight container to keep it fresh.
- Make a large batch and portion it out for a quick snack all week long.

Greek Yogurt with Sliced Kiwi and Chia Seeds

This refreshing snack combines the creamy texture of Greek yogurt with the tangy sweetness of kiwi and the nutritional boost of chia seeds.

Estimated Meal Time: 5 minutes

Ingredients:

- 1/2 cup plain Greek yogurt (lactose-free if needed)
- 1 kiwi, peeled and sliced
- 1 tbsp chia seeds
- A drizzle of honey (optional)

Cooking Method:

1. Spoon the Greek yogurt into a bowl.
2. Top with sliced kiwi and sprinkle with chia seeds.
3. Drizzle with honey if desired.

Nutritional Facts (per serving):

- Calories: 180 | Protein: 15g | Carbs: 18g | Fat: 6g | Fiber: 5g

Substitution Variations:

- Swap kiwi for strawberries or blueberries if preferred.
- Use almond milk yogurt for a dairy-free option.

Portion Control:

- One serving is 1/2 cup of yogurt with fruit and seeds.

Pro Tips:

- Let the chia seeds sit for a few minutes to absorb some liquid and create a more pudding-like texture.
- You can make this snack ahead of time and store it in the fridge for a quick grab-and-go option.

Sliced Cucumber with Feta and Olive Oil

This simple snack is a delightful combination of crunchy cucumber, creamy feta, and rich olive oil.

Estimated Meal Time: 5 minutes

Ingredients:

- 1/2 cucumber, sliced
- 1/4 cup crumbled feta cheese
- 1 tbsp olive oil
- A pinch of salt and pepper

Cooking Method:

1. Slice the cucumber into thin rounds and arrange them on a plate.
2. Sprinkle with crumbled feta cheese.
3. Drizzle with olive oil and season with salt and pepper.

Nutritional Facts (per serving):

- Calories: 150 | Protein: 5g | Carbs: 7g | Fat: 12g | Fiber: 2g

Substitution Variations:

- Use goat cheese instead of feta for a different flavor.
- Add some fresh herbs like mint or basil for extra freshness.

Portion Control:

- One serving is about 1/2 cucumber with 2 tbsp of feta cheese.

Pro Tips:

- This snack is perfect for meal prep, as the ingredients can be prepped in advance and assembled quickly when needed.
- For a more filling snack, add a handful of olives or some cherry tomatoes.

Hard-Boiled Eggs with Salt and Pepper

Hard-boiled eggs are a classic, protein-packed snack that's quick to make and easy to carry with you.

Estimated Meal Time: 10 minutes

Ingredients:

- 2 large eggs
- Salt and pepper to taste

Cooking Method:

1. Place the eggs in a pot of cold water and bring to a boil.
2. Once boiling, reduce the heat and simmer for 9-10 minutes.
3. Remove the eggs and let them cool before peeling.
4. Sprinkle with salt and pepper to taste.

Nutritional Facts (per serving):

- Calories: 140 | Protein: 12g | Carbs: 2g | Fat: 10g | Fiber: 0g

Substitution Variations:

- Add a sprinkle of paprika or hot sauce for a little kick.
- Pair with low FODMAP veggies for added crunch.

Portion Control:

- One serving is 2 hard-boiled eggs.

Pro Tips:

- To make peeling easier, chill the eggs in ice water after boiling.
- Hard-boiled eggs can be stored in the fridge for up to 5 days.

Banana with Almond Butter

A simple and satisfying snack, this combination of banana and almond butter is sweet, creamy, and full of nutrients.

Estimated Meal Time: 5 minutes

Ingredients:

- 1 banana
- 1 tbsp almond butter

Cooking Method:

1. Slice the banana into rounds.
2. Spread almond butter on top of each slice.

Nutritional Facts (per serving):

- Calories: 220 | Protein: 5g | Carbs: 30g | Fat: 10g | Fiber: 4g

Substitution Variations:

- Use peanut butter or cashew butter if preferred.
- Add a sprinkle of cinnamon or cocoa powder for extra flavor.

Portion Control:

- One serving is one medium banana with 1 tbsp of almond butter.

Pro Tips:

- For extra crunch, top the banana slices with chopped nuts or granola.
- Pre-slice the banana and portion out the almond butter for an easy-to-assemble snack.

Low FODMAP Trail Mix with Dried Cranberries and Pumpkin Seeds

This trail mix is a perfect balance of sweet and savory, with the tartness of cranberries and the crunch of pumpkin seeds.

Estimated Meal Time: 5 minutes

Ingredients:

- 1/4 cup dried cranberries (unsweetened)
- 1/4 cup pumpkin seeds
- 1/4 cup almonds

Cooking Method:

1. Combine the cranberries, pumpkin seeds, and almonds in a small bowl.

Nutritional Facts (per serving):

- Calories: 180 | Protein: 5g | Carbs: 20g | Fat: 12g | Fiber: 3g

Substitution Variations:

- Swap pumpkin seeds for sunflower seeds.
- Add a handful of dark chocolate chips for a treat.

Portion Control:

- One serving is about 1/2 cup of the trail mix.

Pro Tips:

- Store this trail mix in small containers for easy on-the-go snacks.
- Make a larger batch and keep it in the pantry for a quick snack whenever needed.

Rice Crackers with Cheddar Cheese

A simple yet satisfying snack, rice crackers paired with cheddar cheese offer a delicious balance of crunch and creaminess.

Estimated Meal Time: 5 minutes

Ingredients:

- 6-8 rice crackers
- 1 oz cheddar cheese, sliced

Cooking Method:

1. Arrange the rice crackers on a plate.
2. Top with slices of cheddar cheese.

Nutritional Facts (per serving):

- Calories: 200 | Protein: 8g | Carbs: 18g | Fat: 14g | Fiber: 2g

Substitution Variations:

- Swap cheddar for any other low FODMAP cheese, like mozzarella or Swiss.
- Add a few slices of cucumber or tomato on top for extra freshness.

Portion Control:

- One serving is 6-8 crackers with cheese.

Pro Tips:

- Choose brown rice crackers for added fiber.
- For a savory snack, sprinkle with a pinch of herbs or spices.

Each of these low FODMAP-friendly snacks will help you stay energized throughout the day without compromising your digestive health. They're quick to prepare, delicious, and perfect for satisfying cravings between meals!

Desserts

Here are some delightful low FODMAP dessert options that satisfy your sweet cravings while keeping your digestive health in mind. Each treat is simple to make and offers a delicious way to indulge without the discomfort.

Low FODMAP Chocolate Avocado Mousse

A rich and creamy dessert with the perfect balance of chocolatey indulgence and healthy fats from avocado.

Estimated Meal Time: 10 minutes

Ingredients:

- 2 ripe avocados, peeled and pitted
- 1/4 cup unsweetened cocoa powder
- 1/4 cup maple syrup or honey
- 1 tsp vanilla extract
- 1/4 cup almond milk

Cooking Method:

1. In a food processor, combine the avocado, cocoa powder, maple syrup, vanilla, and almond milk.
2. Blend until smooth and creamy.
3. Refrigerate for 30 minutes before serving.
4. Serve chilled, topped with shaved dark chocolate or berries.

Nutritional Facts (per serving):

- Calories: 180 | Protein: 2g | Carbs: 22g | Fat: 12g | Fiber: 7g

Substitution Variations:

- Use coconut milk or oat milk instead of almond milk for a different flavor.
- Add a pinch of sea salt for an enhanced chocolate flavor.

Portion Control:

- One serving is approximately 1/4 cup of mousse.

Pro Tips:

- Make the mousse ahead of time and store in the fridge for a quick and healthy dessert.
- For a sweeter mousse, adjust the sweetness by adding more maple syrup or honey.

Blueberry Almond Chia Pudding

A healthy and refreshing dessert with a burst of blueberry flavor, perfect for a snack or a light dessert.

Estimated Meal Time: 5 minutes (plus 4 hours to set)

Ingredients:

- 1/2 cup chia seeds
- 1 cup almond milk (or any milk of your choice)
- 1/4 cup fresh blueberries
- 1 tbsp maple syrup or honey
- 1/4 tsp vanilla extract

Cooking Method:

1. In a bowl, combine chia seeds, almond milk, maple syrup, and vanilla extract.
2. Stir well and cover the bowl.
3. Refrigerate for at least 4 hours or overnight.
4. Top with fresh blueberries before serving.

Nutritional Facts (per serving):

- Calories: 120 | Protein: 3g | Carbs: 14g | Fat: 7g | Fiber: 6g

Substitution Variations:

- Add a few tablespoons of flaxseeds for an extra boost of fiber.
- Use frozen blueberries if fresh ones aren't available.

Portion Control:

- A 1/2 cup serving is a perfect portion for a light and satisfying dessert.

Pro Tips:

- Make multiple servings ahead of time for an easy grab-and-go treat.

- For added crunch, top with sliced almonds or granola.

Banana and Coconut Milk Popsicles

These creamy popsicles are a perfect way to cool off on a warm day, with the sweet flavor of ripe bananas and coconut milk.

Estimated Meal Time: 5 minutes (plus 4 hours to freeze)

Ingredients:

- 2 ripe bananas
- 1 cup coconut milk
- 1 tbsp honey or maple syrup
- 1/2 tsp vanilla extract

Cooking Method:

1. In a blender, combine the bananas, coconut milk, honey, and vanilla extract.
2. Blend until smooth.
3. Pour the mixture into popsicle molds and freeze for at least 4 hours.
4. Once frozen, run warm water over the outside of the molds to release the popsicles.

Nutritional Facts (per popsicle):

- Calories: 80 | Protein: 1g | Carbs: 21g | Fat: 3g | Fiber: 2g

Substitution Variations:

- Add a handful of berries or mango chunks to the mixture before blending for extra flavor.
- Use almond milk or oat milk if you prefer a different base.

Portion Control:

- One popsicle makes a great snack or dessert for a light treat.

Pro Tips:

- For a tropical twist, add a small amount of pineapple or coconut flakes into the mix.
- Make a double batch and store in the freezer for future cravings.

FODMAP-Friendly Apple Crisp

This warm apple crisp features cinnamon-spiced apples and a crunchy topping, offering comfort without any digestive worries.

Estimated Meal Time: 10 minutes (plus 30 minutes to bake)

Ingredients:

- 4 medium apples, peeled, cored, and sliced
- 1/4 cup rolled oats (gluten-free if needed)
- 1/4 cup almond flour
- 2 tbsp brown sugar or maple syrup
- 1/2 tsp cinnamon
- 2 tbsp butter (or dairy-free butter)

Cooking Method:

1. Preheat the oven to 350°F (175°C).
2. Toss the sliced apples with lemon juice and place them in a baking dish.
3. In a separate bowl, combine oats, almond flour, brown sugar, cinnamon, and butter.
4. Sprinkle the oat mixture over the apples and bake for 25-30 minutes, or until the apples are tender and the topping is golden brown.

Nutritional Facts (per serving):

- Calories: 180 | Protein: 3g | Carbs: 28g | Fat: 7g | Fiber: 5g

Substitution Variations:

- Use pears or peaches in place of apples for a different fruit flavor.
- Swap butter with coconut oil for a dairy-free version.

Portion Control:

- A small 1/2 cup serving is all you need to enjoy this warm, comforting dessert.

Pro Tips:

- Serve with a scoop of lactose-free vanilla ice cream or a dollop of whipped cream for an extra treat.

- For added crunch, sprinkle a few chopped nuts over the top before baking.

Coconut Macaroons

These chewy coconut macaroons are lightly sweetened and perfect for a quick, satisfying dessert with just a few ingredients.

Estimated Meal Time: 10 minutes (plus 15 minutes to bake)

Ingredients:

- 2 1/2 cups unsweetened shredded coconut
- 2 egg whites
- 1/4 cup maple syrup
- 1 tsp vanilla extract
- A pinch of sea salt

Cooking Method:

1. Preheat the oven to 325°F (163°C).
2. In a bowl, whisk the egg whites, maple syrup, vanilla extract, and sea salt together.
3. Stir in the shredded coconut until well combined.
4. Spoon the mixture onto a baking sheet lined with parchment paper and bake for 15-20 minutes, or until golden brown.

Nutritional Facts (per serving):

- Calories: 150 | Protein: 2g | Carbs: 14g | Fat: 10g | Fiber: 3g

Substitution Variations:

- Add a few dark chocolate chips for a chocolatey twist.
- Use honey instead of maple syrup for a different flavor profile.

Portion Control:

- One macaroon is a perfect serving for a small but sweet treat.

Pro Tips:

- Store in an airtight container for up to a week for a quick and easy snack.

- For a lighter version, reduce the amount of maple syrup slightly.

Almond Flour Shortbread Cookies

These delicate, buttery shortbread cookies made with almond flour are the perfect low FODMAP treat to satisfy your sweet tooth.

Estimated Meal Time: 15 minutes (plus 15-20 minutes to bake)

Ingredients:

- 1 1/2 cups almond flour
- 1/4 cup coconut flour
- 1/4 cup butter (or dairy-free butter)
- 2 tbsp maple syrup
- 1/4 tsp vanilla extract
- A pinch of sea salt

Cooking Method:

1. Preheat the oven to 325°F (163°C) and line a baking sheet with parchment paper.
2. In a bowl, combine almond flour, coconut flour, and sea salt.
3. In a separate bowl, whisk together melted butter, maple syrup, and vanilla extract.
4. Add the wet ingredients to the dry ingredients and mix until dough forms.
5. Roll the dough into small balls and flatten them with a fork or your fingers.
6. Bake for 15-20 minutes, or until the cookies are golden brown around the edges.

Nutritional Facts (per serving):

- Calories: 120 | Protein: 3g | Carbs: 5g | Fat: 10g | Fiber: 2g

Substitution Variations:

- Add a small amount of lemon zest or almond extract for extra flavor.
- Swap maple syrup for honey for a different sweetness.

Portion Control:

- One shortbread cookie is a great, satisfying serving.

Pro Tips:

- For extra crunch, sprinkle a little chopped almond or crushed walnuts on top of each cookie before baking.

- These cookies store well in an airtight container for up to a week.

Low FODMAP Strawberry Sorbet

A refreshing and fruity dessert that's naturally sweet and dairy-free, made with just a few simple ingredients.

Estimated Meal Time: 5 minutes (plus 4 hours to freeze)

Ingredients:

- 2 cups fresh or frozen strawberries
- 1/2 cup maple syrup
- 1/4 cup water
- 1 tsp lemon juice

Cooking Method:

1. In a blender, combine strawberries, maple syrup, water, and lemon juice.
2. Blend until smooth and pour the mixture into a shallow container.
3. Freeze for at least 4 hours or until firm.
4. Scoop the sorbet into bowls and serve.

Nutritional Facts (per serving):

- Calories: 80 | Protein: 1g | Carbs: 20g | Fat: 0g | Fiber: 4g

Substitution Variations:

- Swap strawberries for other low FODMAP fruits like blueberries or raspberries.
- Add a splash of lime juice for a zesty twist.

Portion Control:

- One serving is about 1/2 cup of sorbet.

Pro Tips:

- If the sorbet is too firm, let it sit at room temperature for a few minutes before serving.

- Make a double batch and store extra in the freezer for future cravings.

Lemon Coconut Energy Bites

Packed with coconut and a burst of citrus flavor, these energy bites are perfect for a quick snack or a light dessert.

Estimated Meal Time: 10 minutes

Ingredients:

- 1 cup unsweetened shredded coconut
- 1/4 cup almond flour
- 2 tbsp maple syrup
- 1 tbsp lemon zest
- 2 tbsp lemon juice
- 1 tbsp coconut oil

Cooking Method:

1. In a bowl, mix together shredded coconut, almond flour, maple syrup, lemon zest, and lemon juice.
2. Add melted coconut oil and stir until the mixture comes together.
3. Roll the mixture into small balls and place on a parchment-lined tray.
4. Refrigerate for at least 1 hour to firm up.

Nutritional Facts (per serving):

- Calories: 100 | Protein: 2g | Carbs: 8g | Fat: 8g | Fiber: 3g

Substitution Variations:

- Add a handful of chopped almonds or cashews for a nutty crunch.
- Use orange zest and juice for a different citrus flavor.

Portion Control:

- One energy bite is a perfect serving.

Pro Tips:

- Store these bites in an airtight container for up to a week.

- For added sweetness, drizzle with a little extra maple syrup before refrigerating.

Low FODMAP Oatmeal Raisin Cookies

A comforting and classic treat made with oats, raisins, and warm spices, perfect for a satisfying dessert.

Estimated Meal Time: 15 minutes (plus 12-15 minutes to bake)

Ingredients:

- 1 1/2 cups rolled oats (gluten-free if needed)
- 1/4 cup almond flour
- 1/2 cup raisins
- 1/4 cup maple syrup
- 1/4 cup butter (or dairy-free butter)
- 1/2 tsp cinnamon
- 1/4 tsp vanilla extract

Cooking Method:

1. Put parchment paper on a baking pan and preheat the oven to 350°F (175°C).
2. In a bowl, combine oats, almond flour, cinnamon, and raisins.
3. In a separate bowl, mix melted butter, maple syrup, and vanilla extract.
4. Add the wet ingredients to the dry ingredients and stir until the dough forms.
5. Drop spoonfuls of dough onto the baking sheet and flatten them slightly.
6. Bake for 12-15 minutes, or until the cookies are golden brown.

Nutritional Facts (per serving):

- Calories: 160 | Protein: 3g | Carbs: 22g | Fat: 7g | Fiber: 3g

Substitution Variations:

- Use dried cranberries instead of raisins for a tangy twist.

- Add a small handful of walnuts or pecans for added crunch.

Portion Control:

- One cookie is a satisfying portion for a sweet snack.

Pro Tips:

- After a few minutes of cooling on the baking sheet, move the cookies to a wire rack.
- These cookies keep well in an airtight container for up to 5 days.

Baked Cinnamon Apples with Walnuts

A warm, comforting dessert that combines the natural sweetness of apples with cinnamon and crunchy walnuts.

Estimated Meal Time: 10 minutes (plus 20-25 minutes to bake)

Ingredients:

- 4 medium apples, cored
- 1/4 cup chopped walnuts
- 1 tbsp maple syrup
- 1 tsp cinnamon
- 1 tbsp butter (or dairy-free butter)

Cooking Method:

1. Preheat the oven to 350°F (175°C).
2. Core the apples and place them in a baking dish.
3. In a small bowl, combine chopped walnuts, maple syrup, cinnamon, and melted butter.
4. Stuff the apples with the walnut mixture and place a little butter on top of each apple.
5. Bake for 20-25 minutes, or until the apples are tender.

Nutritional Facts (per serving):

- Calories: 170 | Protein: 3g | Carbs: 22g | Fat: 10g | Fiber: 4g

Substitution Variations:

- Add raisins or dried cranberries for extra sweetness.

- Use pecans or almonds instead of walnuts for a different flavor.

Portion Control:

- One baked apple is a great portion for a warm and comforting dessert.

Pro Tips:

- Serve with a dollop of lactose-free whipped cream or vanilla ice cream for an extra treat.
- These apples can be made ahead of time and reheated before serving.

These low FODMAP desserts are delicious, easy to make, and offer a perfect balance of sweetness and digestible ingredients. Enjoy them as part of a well-rounded, gut-friendly diet!

Chapter 6

Dining Out and Socializing on the Low FODMAP Diet

Socializing and dining out while following the Low FODMAP diet may seem challenging at first, but with a little preparation and confidence, you can navigate meals and social events with ease. This chapter will offer practical strategies and tips to help you confidently enjoy dining out, attending social gatherings, and managing holiday meals while staying true to your Low FODMAP lifestyle.

Navigating Menus:

Tips for Finding Low-FODMAP Options at Restaurants

Dining out can feel intimidating when you're following a restrictive diet, but many restaurants are becoming more accommodating to special dietary needs. Here are some tips for finding Low FODMAP-friendly options:

1. **Do Your Research:** Many restaurants now offer their menus online. Take a few minutes to browse and check for items that fit your dietary needs. Look for meals that are simple and contain whole, unprocessed ingredients like grilled meats, seafood, salads, or vegetables. Avoid dishes that are likely to have high FODMAP ingredients like garlic, onions, and cream-based sauces.

2. **Choose Grilled or Roasted Dishes:** Opt for grilled or roasted meat and vegetable options, as these are less likely to be prepared with high FODMAP ingredients. For example, grilled chicken, fish, or steak paired with a simple side salad or baked potato is often a safe choice.

3. **Ask for Modifications:** Don't hesitate to ask the server to modify your dish. Most restaurants are willing to accommodate special requests, such as omitting garlic, onions, or sauces. You could ask for the sauce on the side or request that your dish be prepared with olive oil instead of butter.

4. **Stick to Simple, Whole Foods:** If you're unsure about the ingredients in a dish, stick to something simple like grilled meat or fish with steamed vegetables, rice, or potatoes. It's a safe bet that won't include hidden high FODMAP ingredients.

5. **Ask Questions:** If you're in doubt, don't hesitate to ask the server about specific ingredients in a dish. You can inquire if the restaurant uses garlic, onion, or other high FODMAP ingredients in their cooking. Many servers are trained to assist with dietary questions, especially when it comes to popular diets like Low FODMAP.

Communicating Dietary Needs:

Explaining the Diet to Servers, Friends, and Family

One of the biggest challenges when dining out or socializing is effectively communicating your dietary needs. Whether you're at a restaurant or gathering with friends and family, here are some strategies to help you explain your Low FODMAP needs confidently and politely:

1. **Be Clear and Direct with Servers:** When ordering at a restaurant, it's helpful to briefly explain your dietary needs. A simple way to start is by saying, "I follow a Low FODMAP diet for digestive health, which means I need to avoid certain foods like garlic, onions, and high-fiber ingredients." Most servers will appreciate the clarity and will do their best to accommodate your needs.

2. **Request Simple Modifications:** If you're comfortable, provide the server with specific modifications, such as, "Could you please prepare my dish without garlic or onions?" This ensures that your meal is prepared in a way that meets your requirements.

3. **Talk to Friends and Family in Advance:** If you're attending a gathering or party, let your hosts know ahead of time about your dietary needs. You can say, "I'm on a special diet to manage my digestive health, so I avoid certain foods like garlic, onions, and dairy. I'd be happy to bring my own dish or help with the meal planning to ensure I can enjoy the meal."

4. **Be Understanding:** Sometimes people might not be familiar with the Low FODMAP diet, and that's okay. Be patient when explaining your dietary needs. Offer suggestions or resources to make it easier for others to accommodate your requirements, such as sharing a recipe or a list of Low FODMAP foods.

5. **Use a Diet Card:** If you feel uncomfortable explaining your dietary needs each time, consider carrying a small diet card that explains what you can and cannot eat. This can be handed to a server or host to make communication easier and ensure they understand your restrictions.

Handling Social Gatherings:

Strategies for Holidays, Parties, and Events

Attending social events like holidays, parties, or gatherings with friends and family can present unique challenges when following the Low FODMAP diet. However, with a little planning, you can still enjoy these occasions without feeling restricted. Here's how:

1. **Bring Your Own Food:** If you're unsure about what will be available at a party or gathering, bring a dish to share that aligns with your dietary needs. This way, you'll have something safe to eat and others can enjoy it too. Dishes like a Low FODMAP-friendly salad, grilled vegetables, or a simple protein like chicken or fish are great options.

2. **Offer to Contribute:** If the host is preparing a large meal, offer to contribute a Low FODMAP dish that everyone can enjoy. This way, you know you'll have something to eat, and your friends or family will likely appreciate the thoughtfulness.

3. **Practice Portion Control:** If you're at a party where the food options are limited or contain high FODMAP ingredients, try to fill your plate with smaller portions of what is available. You can focus on fruits, vegetables, and proteins that are within the Low FODMAP guidelines, and supplement with your own dish if needed.

4. **Stay Calm and Confident:** If you find yourself at a holiday or social gathering where it's difficult to avoid high FODMAP foods, stay calm. Politely decline foods you cannot eat and explain that you follow a special diet. Most people will be understanding once they know you're prioritizing your health.

5. **Enjoy the Experience:** Socializing isn't just about the food. Focus on the company, conversation, and other aspects of the event. Remind yourself that you're taking care of your health, and that your choices will help you feel better and enjoy life more fully in the long run.

Dining out and socializing on the Low FODMAP diet may require some additional effort, but it's entirely possible to navigate these situations with confidence. By planning ahead, communicating clearly, and finding creative solutions, you can continue to enjoy meals, gatherings, and holidays without feeling left out. Remember, the key is to be proactive, stay positive, and prioritize your well-being. With practice, you'll find that sticking to your Low FODMAP diet can be an empowering experience, helping you take control of your health while still enjoying life's social moments.

Chapter 7

Troubleshooting and Staying on Track

Following the Low FODMAP diet can bring significant benefits for digestive health, but it's not always a smooth journey. You may encounter challenges along the way, whether it's an accidental FODMAP intake, persistent symptoms, or moments when motivation wanes. In this chapter, we'll address some of the common hurdles people face on the Low FODMAP diet and provide practical solutions to help you stay on track and feel your best.

Common Challenges: Dealing with Accidental FODMAP Intake

Accidents happen, and sometimes we may unknowingly consume foods that contain high levels of FODMAPs. This can be frustrating, but it's important to handle these situations with patience and understanding. Here are some ways to manage accidental intake:

1. **Don't Panic:** If you accidentally eat a high FODMAP food, remember that one slip-up is not the end of the world. It's important to stay calm and not let it derail your progress. The body may take a little time to react, so just be mindful of your symptoms over the next few hours.

2. **Stay Hydrated:** Drinking plenty of water after an accidental FODMAP intake can help flush your system and support digestion. Staying hydrated is key when managing any digestive upset.

3. **Rest and Relax:** Stress can exacerbate digestive symptoms, so it's important to relax if you've accidentally consumed a high FODMAP food. Take it easy, rest, and let your body process the food.

4. **Track Your Intake:** Keep a food diary to track what you eat and any symptoms that arise. This will help you pinpoint any triggers and avoid making the same mistake in the future. It's also a helpful way to stay on top of your progress and catch any potential issues early.

5. **Learn from the Experience:** Instead of feeling discouraged, use the experience as an opportunity to learn more about your body and how it reacts to certain foods. Over time, you'll become more attuned to what you can and cannot tolerate.

What to Do When Symptoms Persist: Adjusting the Diet and Seeking Professional Help

Even after following the Low FODMAP diet, it's possible that some symptoms may persist. This can be frustrating, but there are steps you can take to adjust and seek the help you need:

1. **Revisit the Elimination Phase:** If symptoms persist despite following the diet, consider revisiting the elimination phase. Ensure you are strictly avoiding all high FODMAP foods and that you're not unknowingly consuming them. Sometimes, people inadvertently reintroduce high FODMAP foods without realizing it, which can hinder progress.

2. **Track Symptoms and Foods:** Keep a detailed record of the foods you're eating and any symptoms you experience. This will help you identify patterns and possible triggers. Even small amounts of high FODMAP foods can cause issues, so be thorough in tracking your meals and symptoms.

3. **Consider a Food Sensitivity Test:** In some cases, you may have sensitivities to other foods that are not included in the Low FODMAP diet. Consider consulting with a healthcare professional for food sensitivity testing to rule out any other potential triggers.

4. **Consult a Dietitian or Healthcare Provider:** If symptoms persist despite following the diet, it may be time to seek help from a registered dietitian or healthcare provider who specializes in the Low FODMAP diet. They can help you adjust your diet, recommend additional treatments, and ensure you're on the right track. A dietitian can also help with transitioning back to a regular diet after completing the elimination and reintroduction phases.

5. **Be Patient and Persistent:** The Low FODMAP diet is a process, and it may take time to see results. If symptoms continue, be patient with yourself and continue working with a professional to fine-tune your approach. Healing your gut takes time, and the effort you're putting in now will pay off in the long run.

Staying Motivated: Tips to Maintain a Positive Mindset and Long-Term Success

Staying motivated on the Low FODMAP diet can sometimes be challenging, especially when you face setbacks or feel like progress is slow. However, maintaining a positive mindset is key to long-term success. Here are some tips to help you stay motivated:

1. **Set Small, Achievable Goals:** Focus on small milestones, such as trying a new Low FODMAP recipe or going a week without experiencing digestive issues. Celebrate your successes, no matter how small they may seem. Each step forward is a victory!

2. **Stay Connected with Support:** Whether it's through online communities, social media groups, or friends who understand your journey, staying connected with others who are following the Low FODMAP diet can provide encouragement and accountability. Share your struggles and successes, and offer support to others as well.

3. **Focus on the Benefits:** Remind yourself of the positive changes that following the Low FODMAP diet brings to your health. If you're experiencing fewer digestive issues, improved energy levels, or better overall well-being, focus on these improvements to stay motivated. Keep a list of the benefits you've experienced as a reminder of why you're doing this.

4. **Find Joy in Cooking:** If preparing meals feels like a chore, try to make it fun by experimenting with new Low FODMAP recipes or cooking techniques. The more you enjoy the process, the more likely you'll stick to your dietary plan.

5. **Don't Be Too Hard on Yourself:** It's natural to feel frustrated at times, especially if you're struggling with persistent symptoms or missing certain foods. But remember, the Low FODMAP diet is a tool to help you manage your digestive health—it's not about perfection. Give yourself grace and allow yourself the space to learn and grow through this process.

6. **Practice Self-Care:** Your well-being isn't just about food. Incorporate other forms of self-care, like exercise, relaxation, and spending time with loved ones, into your routine. Taking care of your overall health will help you stay grounded and focused on your goals.

7. **Remember Your Why:** Take a moment to reflect on why you started the Low FODMAP diet in the first place. Whether it's to manage digestive issues, improve energy, or simply feel better overall, keeping your "why" in mind can give you the strength to keep going when times get tough.

Following the Low FODMAP diet may come with challenges, but with the right mindset and support, you can overcome any obstacles that arise. By staying patient, adjusting as needed, and maintaining motivation, you'll be well on your way to achieving long-term success. Remember that you're not alone on this journey—there's a community of people who understand what you're going through, and there are plenty of resources to support you. Stay focused, keep experimenting with new recipes, and take pride in the progress you make, no matter how small.

Chapter 8

Long-Term Strategies for Gut Health

While the Low FODMAP diet is an excellent tool for managing digestive issues, it's just one piece of the puzzle when it comes to long-term gut health. Maintaining a healthy gut requires a holistic approach that incorporates not only dietary changes but also other factors like stress management, exercise, and daily lifestyle choices. In this chapter, we'll explore strategies that can help you support your gut health in the long run and ensure that your digestive system stays happy and healthy for years to come.

Beyond FODMAPs: Incorporating Other Gut-Healthy Practices

The Low FODMAP diet is a great starting point, but it's important to view it as part of a broader strategy for maintaining gut health. Once you've successfully navigated the diet and have learned which foods work best for your body, it's time to integrate other gut-friendly practices into your daily routine. Here are a few additional habits that can promote a balanced, thriving gut:

1. **Eat a Variety of Whole, Unprocessed Foods:** In addition to the Low FODMAP foods you've incorporated into your diet, aim to eat a wide range of whole, nutrient-dense foods. Include plenty of fruits, vegetables (that are within your tolerance), whole grains, lean proteins, and healthy fats. A diverse diet provides your gut with the variety it needs to maintain a healthy balance of gut bacteria.

2. **Incorporate Fermented Foods:** Fermented foods are rich in probiotics, which can support the growth of beneficial bacteria in your gut. Consider adding foods like yogurt (low lactose, if necessary), kimchi, sauerkraut, kefir, and miso to your meals. These foods can help strengthen your gut microbiome, which plays a crucial role in digestion and overall health.

3. **Hydrate Well:** Drinking plenty of water throughout the day supports digestion and helps move food and waste through your system. Aim for about 8 cups of water daily, or more if you're physically active. Staying hydrated can also help prevent constipation and promote a healthy gut lining.

4. **Mindful Eating:** Take time to eat slowly and mindfully, paying attention to your body's hunger and fullness cues. This practice helps your digestive system function more efficiently, as it allows your body to fully process food without the stress of overeating. Avoid eating on the go, as it can lead to indigestion and bloating.

The Role of Stress Management: Techniques for Better Digestion

Stress is one of the most significant factors that can impact gut health. It can disrupt the balance of bacteria in your gut, slow digestion, and even lead to symptoms like bloating, gas, and discomfort. Managing stress is an essential part of maintaining long-term digestive health. Here are some techniques to help you manage stress and support your gut:

1. **Mindfulness and Meditation:** Practicing mindfulness can help calm your mind and reduce stress. Try setting aside a few minutes each day to meditate, focusing on your breath and grounding yourself in the present moment. Meditation can activate the parasympathetic nervous system, which helps your body relax and encourages better digestion.

2. **Yoga and Deep Breathing:** Yoga is an excellent way to reduce stress and promote better digestion. Many yoga poses are designed to relieve tension in the abdominal area and encourage movement

through the digestive tract. Deep breathing exercises, such as diaphragmatic breathing, can also stimulate your digestive system and promote relaxation.

3. **Journaling:** Writing down your thoughts and feelings can help you process stress and release pent-up emotions. Journaling can be a therapeutic way to reflect on your day and ease any anxiety that may be affecting your gut. It's also a helpful tool for tracking any emotional triggers that may be linked to digestive symptoms.

4. **Therapy and Counseling:** If stress is overwhelming and affecting your daily life, consider talking to a therapist or counselor. Cognitive-behavioral therapy (CBT) and other forms of therapy can help you develop healthy coping strategies for managing stress and improving your emotional well-being, which in turn supports better gut health.

Exercise and Physical Activity: How Movement Supports Digestion

Exercise isn't just good for your overall health—it's also essential for maintaining a healthy gut. Regular physical activity supports digestion by improving circulation, reducing stress, and promoting the movement of food through your digestive tract. Here's how exercise can benefit your gut:

1. **Improved Gut Motility:** Physical activity helps stimulate the muscles in the digestive tract, which can improve motility and prevent constipation. This can lead to more regular bowel movements and less bloating.

2. **Reduced Inflammation:** Regular exercise helps reduce inflammation in the body, including the gut. Inflammation is a common factor in digestive issues, and reducing it can help promote better digestion and overall gut health.

3. **Better Stress Management:** Exercise is one of the best ways to manage stress. Whether it's a brisk walk, a jog, a yoga class, or a strength-training session, physical activity releases endorphins, which are natural mood boosters that help combat the negative effects of stress on your gut.

4. **Improved Microbiome Health:** Studies have shown that regular physical activity can help improve the diversity of your gut microbiome, which is important for overall gut health. A diverse microbiome is linked to better digestion, stronger immunity, and improved mental health.

5. **Choose Activities You Enjoy:** The key to sticking with an exercise routine is finding something you enjoy. Whether it's dancing, swimming, hiking, or simply walking your dog, choose activities that make you feel good. Consistency is important, so aim for at least 30 minutes of moderate exercise most days of the week.

Other Gut-Friendly Practices to Integrate into Daily Life

In addition to dietary changes, stress management, and exercise, there are other daily practices that can support long-term gut health:

1. **Get Enough Sleep:** Sleep is essential for overall health, including gut health. Aim for 7-9 hours of quality sleep each night. Poor sleep can disrupt the gut microbiome and contribute to digestive issues, so make sleep a priority.

2. **Avoid Smoking and Limit Alcohol:** Smoking and excessive alcohol consumption can harm the gut lining and lead to digestive problems. If possible, quit smoking and limit alcohol intake to support your gut health.

3. **Stay Socially Connected:** Having strong social connections and support networks can help reduce stress and improve mental well-being. Surround yourself with positive, understanding people who support your health journey.

4. **Listen to Your Body:** Finally, always listen to your body. Pay attention to how foods, activities, and lifestyle choices make you feel. This awareness will help you make adjustments to maintain optimal gut health in the long term.

Achieving and maintaining long-term gut health requires more than just following a specific diet. By adopting a holistic approach that includes stress management, exercise, a balanced diet, and mindful living, you can promote a healthy gut for years to come. Be patient with yourself, and remember that small changes over time can lead to significant improvements. Stay consistent, listen to your body, and take pride in the steps you're taking to prioritize your gut health. Your digestive system—and your overall well-being—will thank you for it.

Chapter 9

FAQs About the Low FODMAP Diet

The Low FODMAP diet is a powerful tool for managing digestive issues like IBS, but it can raise many questions. In this chapter, we'll address some of the most common concerns and provide clear, evidence-based answers to help you navigate the diet confidently.

1. Can I ever eat high-FODMAP foods again?

Yes, after completing the elimination phase of the Low FODMAP diet, the goal is to reintroduce high-FODMAP foods gradually to identify which ones you can tolerate. The reintroduction phase allows you to test specific foods and determine your individual tolerance levels. Some people may find they can tolerate certain high-FODMAP foods in small amounts, while others may need to avoid them long-term.

It's important to work with a healthcare professional, such as a dietitian, during this phase to ensure you're reintroducing foods properly and maintaining a balanced, nutritious diet.

2. How do I handle cravings for restricted foods?

Cravings for high-FODMAP foods are normal, especially during the early stages of the diet. Here are some strategies to manage cravings:

- **Find Substitutes:** Look for low-FODMAP alternatives to your favorite high-FODMAP foods. For example, if you're craving pasta, try gluten-free or rice-based pasta. If you're missing dairy, try lactose-free products or dairy-free alternatives like almond milk or coconut yogurt.

- **Satisfy Your Taste Buds:** Focus on enhancing the flavors of low-FODMAP foods. Use herbs, spices, and citrus to add variety to your meals. You might be surprised at how satisfying low-FODMAP versions of your favorite foods can be!

- **Stay Distracted:** Engage in activities you enjoy, like taking a walk, reading, or spending time with friends, to keep your mind off cravings. Sometimes, cravings are more about habit than actual hunger.

- **Give Yourself Time:** It may take time for your body to adjust, but as you continue on the Low FODMAP diet, your cravings will likely decrease. Be patient with yourself and trust that your body will adapt to your new eating habits.

3. Is the Low FODMAP diet safe for children?

The Low FODMAP diet can be helpful for children with digestive issues like IBS, but it should be followed with care and under the guidance of a pediatric dietitian. Children have different nutritional needs compared to adults, and a restrictive diet may lead to nutrient deficiencies if not properly managed. A dietitian will help ensure that the diet is balanced and appropriate for a child's growth and development.

In some cases, the Low FODMAP diet may not be necessary for children with digestive problems. A healthcare professional will help assess whether the diet is the best approach or if other treatments might be more appropriate.

4. Is the Low FODMAP diet safe during pregnancy?

The Low FODMAP diet is generally considered safe during pregnancy, but it should be approached carefully. Pregnancy comes with specific nutritional requirements, and the Low FODMAP diet could limit some foods that are important for both the mother and baby. It is essential to work with a healthcare provider or dietitian to ensure that the diet is nutritionally balanced and meets the needs of both the mother and the developing baby.

In some cases, doctors may recommend modifications or alternative treatments if the Low FODMAP diet is too restrictive. Your healthcare provider will help you determine the best course of action to maintain gut health while supporting a healthy pregnancy.

5. Can I follow the Low FODMAP diet long-term?

The Low FODMAP diet is not intended to be followed long-term. The goal of the diet is to identify trigger foods and help you manage symptoms. After completing the elimination and reintroduction phases, most people are able to reintroduce many high-FODMAP foods back into their diet in moderation, depending on their tolerance levels.

In the long term, your focus should be on maintaining a balanced, diverse diet that includes a variety of foods, while avoiding only the high-FODMAP foods that you cannot tolerate. It's important to work with a dietitian to ensure your diet is balanced and meets all of your nutritional needs.

6. Will the Low FODMAP diet work for everyone with digestive issues?

While the Low FODMAP diet has been proven effective for many people with IBS and other digestive issues, it's not a one-size-fits-all solution. It's possible that the diet may not address all digestive symptoms, particularly if other conditions, such as celiac disease, inflammatory bowel disease (IBD), or food allergies, are present.

If the Low FODMAP diet doesn't seem to be improving symptoms, it's important to seek guidance from a healthcare professional who can help determine the underlying cause of digestive issues and recommend alternative treatments or diets.

7. How long do I need to stay on the elimination phase?

The elimination phase typically lasts for 4-6 weeks, during which you avoid all high-FODMAP foods. This period allows your digestive system to reset and helps determine if the Low FODMAP diet is effective in reducing symptoms. However, the length of time you should stay on the elimination phase may vary based on individual needs and the advice of your healthcare provider.

If you're unsure about how long to stay in the elimination phase or how to proceed with reintroducing foods, it's best to work with a registered dietitian who specializes in the Low FODMAP diet.

8. How do I manage social situations or dining out on the Low FODMAP diet?

Managing social situations and dining out while on the Low FODMAP diet can be challenging, but with the right strategies, you can enjoy meals with friends and family without feeling stressed or restricted.

- **Be proactive:** When dining out, research the restaurant menu beforehand, and don't be afraid to ask the server about ingredient lists and food preparation methods. Many restaurants are willing to accommodate dietary restrictions if you ask politely.

- **Communicate clearly:** Let your friends, family, and colleagues know about your dietary needs. Having their support can make it easier to navigate social gatherings without feeling like you're missing out.

- **Plan ahead:** If you're going to a party or holiday gathering, offer to bring a dish that you know will be safe for you to eat. This way, you can enjoy the event without worrying about finding suitable options.

9. What should I do if I accidentally eat a high-FODMAP food?

Accidents happen, and it's okay if you occasionally consume a high-FODMAP food by mistake. If this occurs, don't panic. Focus on staying calm and allowing your digestive system time to process the food. It may help to drink plenty of water, take a walk, or engage in relaxation techniques to ease any discomfort.

If symptoms are severe or persistent, reach out to your healthcare provider for guidance. They can help you manage the situation and offer advice on adjusting your diet if necessary.

10. Can I drink alcohol on the Low FODMAP diet?

Alcohol can be tricky on the Low FODMAP diet, as many alcoholic drinks contain high-FODMAP ingredients or can irritate the digestive system. While some alcoholic beverages, such as wine and spirits, are generally considered low-FODMAP in moderation, it's important to keep track of how alcohol affects your symptoms.

Be mindful of mixers, as many cocktails contain high-FODMAP ingredients like fruit juices, syrups, or soda. It's best to stick to simple drinks and limit alcohol intake to avoid exacerbating digestive issues.

The Low FODMAP diet is a powerful tool for managing digestive discomfort, but it can raise many questions. Whether you're wondering about cravings, navigating social situations, or considering long-term use, it's important to approach the diet with knowledge and support. Remember, this diet isn't meant to be restrictive forever, and with the right approach, you can enjoy a balanced and fulfilling lifestyle while managing your digestive health.

Chapter 10

A 4-Week Low FODMAP Meal Plan

Here's a more detailed 4-week meal plan, broken down for each day of the week, providing a simple yet balanced approach to following the Low FODMAP diet. Each day features breakfast, lunch, dinner, and snacks, with a grocery shopping list for each week.

Week 1

Day 1

- **Breakfast**: Scrambled Eggs with Spinach and Tomatoes
- **Lunch**: Grilled Chicken Salad (Mixed greens, cucumber, carrots, olive oil, and lemon dressing)
- **Dinner**: Baked Salmon with Roasted Vegetables (Potatoes, carrots, green beans)
- **Snack**: Carrot Sticks with Hummus

Day 2

- **Breakfast**: Blueberry Chia Pudding (Chia seeds, almond milk, blueberries)
- **Lunch**: Low FODMAP Quinoa Salad (Quinoa, roasted zucchini, carrots, lemon-olive oil dressing)
- **Dinner**: Chicken Stir-Fry (Bell peppers, zucchini, spinach, garlic-infused oil)
- **Snack**: Low FODMAP Energy Balls

Day 3

- **Breakfast**: Rice Cakes with Peanut Butter and Banana
- **Lunch**: Turkey Lettuce Wraps (Turkey slices, cucumber, mustard wrapped in lettuce)
- **Dinner**: Low FODMAP Meatballs with Zucchini Noodles (Homemade meatballs, tomato sauce)
- **Snack**: Lactose-Free Yogurt with Strawberries

Day 4

- **Breakfast**: Scrambled Eggs with Spinach and Tomatoes
- **Lunch**: Grilled Chicken Salad
- **Dinner**: Chicken Stir-Fry
- **Snack**: Carrot Sticks with Hummus

Day 5

- **Breakfast**: Blueberry Chia Pudding
- **Lunch**: Low FODMAP Quinoa Salad
- **Dinner**: Baked Salmon with Roasted Vegetables
- **Snack**: Low FODMAP Energy Balls

Day 6

- **Breakfast**: Rice Cakes with Peanut Butter and Banana
- **Lunch**: Turkey Lettuce Wraps
- **Dinner**: Low FODMAP Meatballs with Zucchini Noodles
- **Snack**: Lactose-Free Yogurt with Strawberries

Day 7

- **Breakfast**: Scrambled Eggs with Spinach and Tomatoes
- **Lunch**: Grilled Chicken Salad
- **Dinner**: Baked Salmon with Roasted Vegetables
- **Snack**: Carrot Sticks with Hummus

Grocery Shopping List for Week 1

- Eggs, fresh spinach, cherry tomatoes, blueberries, chia seeds, almond milk, rice cakes, peanut butter, bananas, chicken breast, mixed greens, cucumbers, carrots, quinoa, zucchini, lettuce, salmon, potatoes, green beans, ground beef, olive oil, mustard, lactose-free yogurt.

Week 2

Day 1

- **Breakfast**: Low FODMAP Overnight Oats (Oats, almond milk, chia seeds, blueberries)
- **Lunch**: Grilled Chicken and Avocado Salad (Mixed greens, avocado, tomatoes, lemon vinaigrette)
- **Dinner**: Baked Cod with Mashed Potatoes and Steamed Green Beans
- **Snack**: Rice Cakes with Almond Butter

Day 2

- **Breakfast**: Spinach and Feta Omelette
- **Lunch**: FODMAP-Friendly Veggie Wraps (Roasted veggies, hummus, spinach, whole wheat wrap)
- **Dinner**: Low FODMAP Veggie Stir-Fry (Bell peppers, zucchini, spinach, garlic-infused oil)
- **Snack**: Greek Yogurt with Blueberries

Day 3

- **Breakfast**: Smoothie with Spinach and Strawberries (Spinach, strawberries, almond milk, protein powder)
- **Lunch**: Tuna Salad Lettuce Wraps (Tuna, olive oil, lemon juice wrapped in lettuce)
- **Dinner**: Grilled Shrimp with Rice and Steamed Broccoli

- **Snack**: Low FODMAP Protein Bar

Day 4

- **Breakfast**: Low FODMAP Overnight Oats
- **Lunch**: Grilled Chicken and Avocado Salad
- **Dinner**: Baked Cod with Mashed Potatoes and Steamed Green Beans
- **Snack**: Rice Cakes with Almond Butter

Day 5

- **Breakfast**: Spinach and Feta Omelette
- **Lunch**: FODMAP-Friendly Veggie Wraps
- **Dinner**: Low FODMAP Veggie Stir-Fry
- **Snack**: Greek Yogurt with Blueberries

Day 6

- **Breakfast**: Smoothie with Spinach and Strawberries
- **Lunch**: Tuna Salad Lettuce Wraps
- **Dinner**: Grilled Shrimp with Rice and Steamed Broccoli
- **Snack**: Low FODMAP Protein Bar

Day 7

- **Breakfast**: Low FODMAP Overnight Oats
- **Lunch**: Grilled Chicken and Avocado Salad
- **Dinner**: Baked Cod with Mashed Potatoes and Steamed Green Beans
- **Snack**: Rice Cakes with Almond Butter

Grocery Shopping List for Week 2

- Oats, almond milk, chia seeds, fresh spinach, feta cheese, strawberries, chicken breast, avocados, tomatoes, mixed greens, whole wheat wraps, tuna, cod fillets, potatoes, broccoli, shrimp, rice, Greek yogurt.

Week 3

Day 1

- **Breakfast**: Low FODMAP Pancakes (Almond flour, berries, maple syrup)
- **Lunch**: Chicken and Quinoa Bowl (Chicken, quinoa, spinach, bell peppers, lemon dressing)
- **Dinner**: Grilled Salmon with Sweet Potato
- **Snack**: Low FODMAP Popcorn

Day 2

- **Breakfast**: Avocado Toast on Gluten-Free Bread (Mashed avocado, lemon, gluten-free bread)
- **Lunch**: Turkey and Swiss Lettuce Wraps (Turkey, Swiss cheese, lettuce, mustard)
- **Dinner**: Beef Stir-Fry with Vegetables (Beef, bell peppers, zucchini, carrots, garlic-infused oil)
- **Snack**: Banana with Almond Butter

Day 3

- **Breakfast**: Egg and Veggie Scramble (Eggs, bell peppers, spinach, tomatoes)
- **Lunch**: Chicken and Quinoa Bowl
- **Dinner**: Low FODMAP Chicken Curry (Chicken, coconut milk, rice, sautéed veggies)
- **Snack**: Rice Cakes with Cottage Cheese

Day 4

- **Breakfast**: Low FODMAP Pancakes
- **Lunch**: Turkey and Swiss Lettuce Wraps
- **Dinner**: Beef Stir-Fry with Vegetables
- **Snack**: Low FODMAP Popcorn

Day 5

- **Breakfast**: Avocado Toast on Gluten-Free Bread
- **Lunch**: Chicken and Quinoa Bowl
- **Dinner**: Grilled Salmon with Sweet Potato
- **Snack**: Banana with Almond Butter

Day 6

- **Breakfast**: Egg and Veggie Scramble
- **Lunch**: Chicken and Quinoa Bowl
- **Dinner**: Low FODMAP Chicken Curry
- **Snack**: Rice Cakes with Cottage Cheese

Day 7

- **Breakfast**: Low FODMAP Pancakes
- **Lunch**: Turkey and Swiss Lettuce Wraps
- **Dinner**: Beef Stir-Fry with Vegetables
- **Snack**: Low FODMAP Popcorn

Grocery Shopping List for Week 3

- Almond flour, maple syrup, gluten-free bread, eggs, bell peppers, chicken breast, quinoa, Swiss cheese, sweet potatoes, beef, coconut milk, rice, popcorn kernels, cottage cheese, bananas.

Week 4

Day 1

- **Breakfast**: Egg Muffins with Spinach and Feta (Eggs, spinach, feta, bell peppers)
- **Lunch**: Grilled Chicken and Veggie Salad (Mixed greens, cucumbers, tomatoes, lemon vinaigrette)
- **Dinner**: Baked Chicken with Roasted Vegetables (Carrots, potatoes, zucchini)
- **Snack**: Apple with Peanut Butter

Day 2

- **Breakfast**: Greek Yogurt with Berries (Greek yogurt, blueberries, chia seeds)
- **Lunch**: Tuna and Avocado Salad (Tuna, avocado, lettuce, lemon juice)
- **Dinner**: Grilled Pork Chops with Sweet Potato
- **Snack**: Low FODMAP Trail Mix

Day 3

- **Breakfast**: Smoothie with Banana and Peanut Butter
- **Lunch**: Grilled Chicken and Veggie Salad
- **Dinner**: Shrimp Stir-Fry (Bell peppers, zucchini, garlic-infused oil)
- **Snack**: Hard-Boiled Eggs

Day 4

- **Breakfast**: Egg Muffins with Spinach and Feta
- **Lunch**: Tuna and Avocado Salad
- **Dinner**: Baked Chicken with Roasted Vegetables
- **Snack**: Apple with Peanut Butter

Day 5

- **Breakfast**: Greek Yogurt with Berries
- **Lunch**: Grilled Chicken and Veggie Salad
- **Dinner**: Grilled Pork Chops with Sweet Potato
- **Snack**: Low FODMAP Trail Mix

Day 6

- **Breakfast**: Smoothie with Banana and Peanut Butter

- **Lunch**: Grilled Chicken and Veggie Salad

- **Dinner**: Shrimp Stir-Fry

- **Snack**: Hard-Boiled Eggs

Day 7

- **Breakfast**: Egg Muffins with Spinach and Feta

- **Lunch**: Tuna and Avocado Salad

- **Dinner**: Baked Chicken with Roasted Vegetables

- **Snack**: Apple with Peanut Butter

Grocery Shopping List for Week 4

- Spinach, feta cheese, bell peppers, Greek yogurt, chia seeds, bananas, peanut butter, mixed greens, cucumbers, tomatoes, sweet potatoes, pork chops, apples, low FODMAP trail mix.

This 4-week plan is designed to simplify meal planning and help you enjoy a variety of flavors while sticking to a Low FODMAP diet. Feel free to swap meals from different days, as long as you keep the ingredients within the Low FODMAP guidelines.

Conclusion

Embracing Your Journey to Better Gut Health

Congratulations on reaching the end of this guide! You've come a long way, and it's important to take a moment to celebrate the progress you've made. The Low FODMAP diet can be challenging at times, but you've shown dedication and commitment to improving your gut health and overall well-being. Every small step you've taken—whether it's trying a new recipe, adjusting your meals, or learning more about how food affects your body—has brought you closer to achieving your health goals.

Remember, this journey is about more than just managing symptoms. It's about taking control of your digestive health, gaining a deeper understanding of what your body needs, and giving yourself the tools to live a more vibrant, comfortable life. While there may still be challenges ahead, you're equipped with the knowledge and strategies to face them with confidence.

Know that it's okay to take things one day at a time. You don't have to be perfect—what matters most is your ongoing commitment to taking care of yourself. With each choice you make, you're empowering yourself to live your best life.

As you continue with the Low FODMAP diet and integrate these practices into your routine, remember that your health is a journey. You've already taken the first step, and you're on the path to greater well-being. Trust in the process, stay patient with yourself, and celebrate the small victories along the way. You've got this!

Wishing you all the best as you move forward with confidence and strength on your gut-health journey!

9 798304 461184